Prentice Hall Health

Q&A Review

for Home Care Aide

Prentice Hall Health

Q&A Review

Home Care Aide

Maureen Williams, MEd. RN, C
Manager, Staff Development
Hospice and Palliative Care of Metropolitan Washington
Falls Church, Virginia

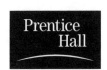

Prentice Hall
Upper Saddle River, New Jersey 07458

Library of Congress Cataloging-in-Publication Data
Williams, Maureen.
   Prentice Hall health Q&A review for
      home care aide/Maureen Williams.
      p. cm.
   Includes bibliographical references and index.
   ISBN 0-13-013142-3
   1. Home health aides—Examinations, questions, etc.
   2. Home care services—Examinations, questions, etc.
   3. Home nursing—Examinations, questions, etc.
I. Title: Health question and answer review for the home
health care.   II. Title.
RA645.3.W547 2000
362.1'4'076—dc21   00-060693

Publisher: Julie Alexander
Executive Editor: Maura Connor
Acquisitions Editor: Barbara Krawiec
Managing Development Editor: Marilyn Meserve
**Director of Production
   and Manufacturing:** Bruce Johnson
Managing Production Editor: Patrick Walsh
Production Editor: Carol Eckhart,
   York Production Services
Production Liaison: Danielle Newhouse
Manufacturing Manager: Ilene Sanford
Creative Director: Marianne Frasco
Cover Design Coordinator: Maria Guglielmo
Cover and Interior Designer: Janice Bielawa
Director of Marketing: Leslie Cavaliere
Marketing Coordinator: Cindy Frederick
Editorial Assistants: Melissa Kerian and
   Mary Ellen Ruitenberg
Composition: York Production Services
Printing and Binding: The Banta Company

Prentice-Hall International (UK) Limited, *London*
Prentice-Hall of Australia Pty. Limited, *Sydney*
Prentice-Hall Canada Inc., *Toronto*
Prentice-Hall Hispanoamericana, S.A., *Mexico*
Prentice-Hall of India Private Limited, *New Delhi*
Prentice-Hall of Japan, Inc., *Tokyo*
Prentice-Hall Singapore Pte. Ltd.
Editora Prentice-Hall do Brasil, Ltda., *Rio de Janeiro*

Notice: It is the intent of the author and publishers that this textbook be used as part of a formal Homemaker/Home Health Aide course taught by a qualified instructor. The Procedures presented here represent accepted practices in the United States. They are not offered as a standard of care. Home health care is to be performed under the authority and guidance of qualified supervisory personnel. It is the reader's responsibility to know and follow local care protocols as provided by the medical advisors directing the system to which he or she belongs. Also, it is the reader's responsibility to stay informed of home health care procedure changes.

The material in this textbook contains the most current information available at the time of publication. However, federal, state and local guidelines concerning clinical practices, including without limitation, those governing infection control and standard precautions, change rapidly. The reader should note, therefore, that new regulations may require changes in some procedures.

It is the responsibility of the reader to familiarize himself or herself with the policies and procedures set by federal, state and local agencies, as well as the institution or agency where the reader is employed. The authors and the publishers of this textbook, and the supplements written to accompany it, disclaim any liability, loss or risk resulting directly or indirectly from the suggested procedures and theory, from any undetected errors, or from the reader's misunderstanding of the text. It is the reader's responsibility to stay informed of any new changes or recommendations made by any federal, state and local agency as well as by his or her employing health care institution or agency.

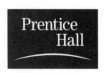
Prentice Hall

10 9 8 7 6 5 4 3 2 1
ISBN 0-13-013142-3

Contents

Preface

The *Prentice Hall Health Q&A Review for Home Care Aide* has been designed to prepare the student for the national home care aide certification examinations. The book provides 1,000 multiple-choice questions, covering the topics most likely to be tested on the examinations.

Following the content of *A Model Curriculum and Teaching Guide for Instruction of the Home Care Aide*, the book is divided into three sections:

Home Care Aide Services: Working with Various Patient Populations
Practical Knowledge and Skills in Home Management
Practical Knowledge and Skills in Personal Care

Sixteen chapters address all areas covered by the national written examination. Topics of unique interest to home care aides are reviewed, including mental health and mental illness; death and dying; working with infants and children; home maintenance and management; food preparation, storage, and safety issues; and assisting with medications.

The correct answers and comprehensive rationales for those answers give students the opportunity to expand their knowledge and understand why answers are correct or incorrect. References following each rationale will direct the user to other resources for more in-depth study. An examlike practice test of 50 questions at the end of the book will give the student a chance to simulate the test-taking experience. The enclosed CD-ROM was designed so that the user can choose to practice questions by topic or through simulated examinations. An audio glossary will provide a review of the definitions and pronunciations of important terms.

Students will find the *Prentice Hall Health Q&A Review for Home Care Aide* to be a valuable tool for review and practice before taking the certification examination.

Maureen Williams

Acknowledgments

Heartfelt thanks are extended to:

My Patrick, for his patience;

Barbara Krawiec, for her encouragement;

Home Care Aides, who have taught me more than I could ever teach them.

Additional thanks to:

Contributor and Reviewer
Lou Ebrite, RN, PhD
Edmond, OK
Professor Emeritus, University of Central Oklahoma

Contributor and Reviewer
Marti Burton, RN, BS
Yukon, OK
Writer and Developer of Custom Health Education Materials

Reviewer
Sulinda Moffett, BSN, MSN, MEd.
Oklahoma City, OK

Introduction

 SUCCESS ACROSS THE BOARDS:
THE PRENTICE HALL HEALTH REVIEW SERIES

Prentice Hall Health is pleased to present *Success Across the Boards,* our new review series. These authoritative texts give you expert help in preparing for certifying examinations. Each title in the series comes with its own technology package, including a CD-ROM and a Companion Website. You will find that this powerful combination of text and media provides you with expert help and guidance for achieving success across the boards.

COMPONENTS OF THE SERIES:

The series is made up of a book and CD-ROM combinations as well as a Companion Website that support the book.

About the Book:

- *Study Questions: Prentice Hall Health Q&A Review for Home Care Aide.* The book has been designed to help the student prepare for the written certification exam. One thousand multiple-choice questions are organized by all the topics covered on the exam and follow the exam format. Working through these questions will help you to assess your strengths and weaknesses in each topic of study. Correct answers and comprehensive rationales are included. All questions are referenced to related textbooks so that you can quickly and easily find resources for more in-depth explanation or study on a specific topic.
- *Practice Exam:* An examlike practice test with 50 questions is included at the end of the book. This test will give you a chance to experience the exam before you actually have to take it. These questions also include correct answers, comprehensive rationales, and references to assist you in determining your strengths, weaknesses, and needs for further study.
- *About the CD-ROM:* A CD-ROM is included in the back of this book. The accompanying CD includes all questions presented in the book plus an audio glossary. Correct answers, comprehensive rationales and references follow all questions. You will receive immediate feedback to identify your strengths and weaknesses in each topic covered. An audio glossary, including over 200 words and definitions, will help you to review the definitions and practice pronunciations of the all-important terms you need to know.

Companion Website for Home Care Aide Review

Visit the Companion Website at **www.prenhall.com/review** for additional practice, information about the exam, and links to related resources. This site was designed as a supplement to this book in the series, and you will want to bookmark it and return frequently for the most current information on your path to success.

CERTIFICATION

The National Association for Home Care (NAHC) sponsors a national certification program for home care aides through its affiliate, HomeCare University. The components of the HomeCare University Program for home care aides include the following:

1. Completion and documentation of a 75-hour training program based on NAHC's *A Model Curriculum and Teaching Guide for the Instruction of the Home Care Aide*
2. Documentation of skills competency utilizing NAHC's *Summary Documentation for Skills Demonstration Checklists*
3. Passing a national written examination.

Since the program began in 1990, over 28,000 home care aides have been certified through this national program, establishing a national standard for preparation of home care aides. The names of all home care aides who successfully complete all three components are placed in the national registry of certified home care aides.

ABOUT THE EXAM

The National Home Care Aide Certification Examination is a written test administered by HomeCare University. The exam is given annually at the National Home Care Aide Service Conference, sponsored by the Home Care Aide Association of America and throughout the United States at local test sites throughout the year.

The examination contains 50 multiple-choice questions selected from the four major sections of the *Model Curriculum:*

Section I (6 questions): Orientation to Homemaker-Home Health Aid Services

Section II (9 questions): Understanding and Working with Various Client Populations

Section III (9 questions): Practical Knowledge and Skills in Home Management

Section IV (26 questions): Practical Knowledge and Skills in Personal Care

Information about the examination and an application may be obtained by contacting HomeCare University, 519 C Street, NE, Washington, DC 20002 (phone: 202-547-7424; fax: 202-547-4322; website: www.nahc.org).

Information about the examination may change, so be sure to obtain current information by contacting HomeCare University.

STUDY TIPS

Review Materials

Choose review materials that contain the information you need to study. Save time by making sure that you aren't studying anything you don't need to. Before the exam, the best study preparation would be to use this Question & Answer Review to identify your strengths and weaknesses. The references at the end of each rationale will direct you to additional resources for more in-depth study.

Set a Study Schedule

Use your time management skills to set a schedule that will help you feel as prepared as you can be. Consider all the relevant factors: the materials you need to study; how many months, weeks, or days until the test date; and how much time you can study each day. If you establish your schedule ahead of time and write it in your date book, you will be much more likely to follow it.

Take Practice Tests

Practice as much as possible, using the questions in this book, on the accompanying CD, and at the companion website. These questions were designed to follow the format of questions that appear on the exam you will take, so the more you practice with these questions, the better prepared you will be on test day.

The printed practice test in the back of the book and the practice tests on the CD will give you a chance to experience the exam before you actually have to take it and will also let you know how you're doing and where you need to do better. For best results, we recommend that you take a practice test 2 to 3 weeks before you are scheduled to take the actual exam. Spend the next weeks targeting the areas in which you performed poorly by reviewing questions in those areas.

Practice under testlike conditions: in a quiet room, with no books or notes to help you, and with a clock telling you when to quit. Try to come as close as you can to duplicating the actual test situation.

TAKING THE EXAMINATION

Prepare Physically

When taking the exam, you need to work efficiently under time pressure. If your body is tired or under stress, you might not think as clearly or perform as well as you usually do. Avoid staying up all night. Get some sleep so that you can wake up rested and alert.

Eating right is also important. The best advice is to eat a light, well-balanced meal before a test. When time is short, grab a quick-energy snack such as a banana, orange juice, or a granola bar.

The Examination Site

The examination site must be located before the required examination time. One suggestion is to find the site and parking facilities the day before the test. Parking fee information should be obtained so that sufficient money can be taken along on the examination day.

Allow plenty of time for travel to the site in case of unexpected mishaps such as traffic snarls. During travel, think positive thoughts (e.g., "My preparation for the exam was thorough, so I'll be able to answer the questions easily"). Maintain a confident attitude to prevent unnecessary stress.

Materials

Be sure to take all required identification materials, registration forms, and any other items required by the testing organization or center. Read information and instructions supplied by the testing organizations thoroughly to be sure you have all necessary materials before the day of the exam.

Read Test Directions

Read the examination directions thoroughly! Because some board examinations have different test sections with different question formats, it is important to be aware of changes in directions. Read each set of directions completely before starting a new section of questions.

Machine-scored tests require that you use a special pencil to fill in a small box on a computerized answer sheet. Use the right pencil (usually a number 2), and mark your answers in the correct space. Neatness counts on these tests, because the computer can misread stray pencil marks or partially erased answers. Periodically, check the answer number against the question number to make sure they match. One question skipped can cause every answer following it to be marked incorrect.

Selecting the Right Answer

Keep in mind that only one answer is correct. First read the stem of the question with each possible choice provided, and eliminate choices that are obviously incorrect. Be cautious about choosing the first answer that *might* be correct; all possibilities should be considered before the final choice is made; the best answer should be selected.

If a question is complicated, try to break it down into small sections that are easy to understand. Pay special attention to qualifiers such as *only* and *except*. For example, negative words in a question can confuse your understanding of what the question asks ("Which of the following is not . . .").

Intelligent Guessing

If you don't know the answer, eliminate the answers that you know or suspect are wrong. Your goal is to narrow down your choices. Here are some questions to ask yourself:

- Is the choice accurate in its own terms? If there's an error in the choice, for example, a term that is incorrectly defined, the answer is wrong.
- Is the choice relevant? An answer may be accurate, but it may not relate to the essence of the question.
- Are there any distractors, such as *always*, *never*, *all*, *none*, or *every*? Qualifiers make it easy to find an exception that makes a choice incorrect.

Mark answers you aren't sure of, and go back to them at the end of the test. Ask yourself whether you would make the same guesses again. Chances are that you will leave your answers alone, but you may notice something that will make you change your mind—a qualifier that affects meaning or a remembered fact that will enable you to answer the question without guessing.

Watch the Clock

Keep track of how much time is left and how you are progressing. Wear a watch, or bring a small clock with you to the test room. A wall clock may be broken, or there may be no clock at all.

Some students are so concerned about time that they rush through the exam and have time left over. In such situations, it's easy to leave early. However, the best approach, is to take your time. Stay until the end so that you can check your answers.

KEYS TO SUCCESS ACROSS THE BOARDS

- Study, review, and practice
- Keep a positive, confident attitude
- Follow all directions on the examination
- Do your best

Good luck!

You are encouraged to visit **http://www.prenhall. com/success** *for additional tips on studying, test taking, and other keys to success. At this state of your education and career, you will find these tips helpful.*

Some of the study and test-taking tips were adapted from Keys to Effective Learning, *Second Edition, by Carol Carter, Joyce Bishop, and Sarah Lyman Kravits.*

References

Foundation for Hospice and Homecare (1990). *A Model Curriculum and Teaching Guide for the Instruction of the Homemaker-Home Health Aide.* Washington, DC: Author.

Marrelli, T. M., & Whittier, S. M. (1996). *Home Health Aide: Guidelines for Care.* Kent Island, MD: Marrelli and Associates, Inc.

Zucker, E. D. (1998). *Being a Homemaker/Home Health Aide*, 5th ed. Upper Saddle River, NJ: Prentice Hall Health.

Home Care Aide Services: Working with Various Patient Populations

1 Communication, Observation, and Rights

chapter objectives

Upon completion of Chapter 1, the student is responsible for the following:

➤ Identify the purpose and organization of a home health agency.

➤ Identify the responsibilities of members of the health care team.

➤ Identify the responsibilities and tasks of the home care aide.

➤ Identify desirable qualities in a home care aide.

➤ Describe types of communication.

➤ Describe subjective and objective reporting.

➤ List techniques of observation.

➤ Define patient rights and responsibilities.

DIRECTIONS
Each of the questions or incomplete statements below is followed by four suggested answers or completions. Select **one answer** that is best in each case.

1. All of the following individuals are members of the health care team except:
   A. nurses
   B. home care aides
   C. administrators
   D. nutritionists

2. Home care aide qualities for success include all of the following except:
   A. timeliness
   B. judgmental attitude
   C. patience
   D. honesty

3. The roles and responsibilities of the home care aide are described in the:
   A. job description
   B. policies and procedures
   C. transfer summary
   D. nursing assessment

4. Which of the following is concerned with restoring function and preventing disability following disease, injury, or loss of a body part?
   A. social worker
   B. physical therapist
   C. physician
   D. nurse

5. Which of the following qualities will ensure success as a home care aide?
   A. You can be trusted.
   B. You try to be courteous.
   C. You are a good listener.
   D. all of the above

6. To understand your roles and expectations as a home care aide, you should rely on:
   A. patients
   B. other home care aides at your agency
   C. nursing supervisor
   D. physician

7. Your patient informs you that she received a bill for your services, and she has questions about this. To whom should you report this information?
   A. supervisor
   B. agency accountant
   C. other home care aides
   D. take care of it yourself

8. Communication among interdisciplinary team members should occur on a regular basis with input from the following:
   A. home care aide
   B. nurse
   C. social worker
   D. all of the above

9. It is very important that you arrive promptly at your patient's home(s) every day unless you are ill. This home care aide quality is an example of:
   A. following directions
   B. accuracy
   C. dependability
   D. efficiency

10. Following your supervisor's instructions exactly and reporting mistakes are examples of the home care aide quality of:
    A. accuracy
    B. timeliness
    C. cleanliness
    D. courtesy

11. Ethics is:
    A. taking pride in your appearance
    B. your job function
    C. a code of rules set up to govern behavior
    D. an exchange of information

12. Do not discuss patient information with:
    A. one patient about another patient
    B. relatives and friends of the patient
    C. your own relatives and friends
    D. All of the above

13. Your fellow home care aide tells you that to save time, she just gives the patient a sponge bath, although a bed bath has been ordered. This is an instance of:
    A. efficiency
    B. negligence
    C. high-quality care
    D. confidentiality

14. While walking up the steps to your patient's home, you trip and fall, scraping your knee and elbow. This is an example of:
    A. carelessness
    B. an incident
    C. neglect
    D. abuse

15. To whom should you report an incident or accident on the job?
    A. supervisor
    B. physician
    C. your family
    D. patient

16. When you say "Good morning" to your patient, you are demonstrating:
    A. verbal communication
    B. nonverbal communication
    C. written communication
    D. body language

17. Body language is a form of which type of communication?
    A. verbal
    B. written
    C. nonverbal
    D. interpretive

18. All of the following are examples of body language except:
    A. facial expressions
    B. touching others
    C. speaking
    D. hand movements

19. To relate and communicate with people, you must:
    A. be courteous
    B. be tactful
    C. be sensitive
    D. all of the above

20. Changes in patient status that should be reported to your nursing supervisor include:
    A. breathing changes
    B. bleeding
    C. pain
    D. all of the above

21. The home care aide participates in the development of the patient's plan of care by:
    A. writing the plan of care
    B. observing and reporting patient status
    C. obtaining physician orders
    D. all of the above

22. When a patient makes a comment about other members of the health care team, the home care aide should:
    A. agree with the patient
    B. speak with the supervisor
    C. encourage the patient to say more
    D. all of the above

23. The home care aide should complete documentation of patient care:
    A. within 1 week
    B. in pencil so that you can erase errors and make corrections
    C. as soon as possible after giving care
    D. only if an incident occurs

24. An example of subjective reporting of patient care is:

    A. Patient said, "I don't feel well today."

    B. Temperature of 101.2°F.

    C. Vomiting green emesis.

    D. none of the above

25. An example of subjective reporting of patient care is:

    A. Patient's buttocks are red.

    B. "Yesterday, Mrs. C. and her landlady were talking in loud voices. I just know they were fighting."

    C. Pulse is 104.

    D. Patient had four bowel movements during visit.

26. Examples of objective reporting include all of the following except:

    A. Patient is OK today.

    B. Patient is breathing 20 times a minute and complains of chest pain.

    C. Patient says she has a pain in her right upper abdomen.

    D. Patient says he sees horses on the ceiling about 30 minutes after taking his pills.

27. Basic guidelines to be used in reporting and recording include:

    A. report all changes in a patient's condition

    B. record observations on a weekly basis

    C. report the events in the order in which they occurred

    D. all except B

28. A key component of the patient's bill of rights is:

    A. the right to have medications paid for

    B. the right to have an active part in establishing the care plan

    C. the right to have housekeepers

    D. the right to abuse the home care aide

29. The home care aide may discuss the patient with:

    A. the nurse supervisor

    B. the patient's neighbor

    C. the patient's brother

    D. the patient's attorney

30. Each of the following is a part of the patient's bill of rights except:

    A. the right to privacy

    B. the right to refuse care

    C. the right to be treated with respect

    D. the right to yell at workers

31. The home care aide's primary function is to:

    A. provide basic personal care

    B. administer tube feedings

    C. administer medications

    D. contact the physician for orders

32. Medicare and Medicaid are health insurance payment plans primarily for those of low income and:

    A. veterans

    B. the elderly

    C. wealthy people

    D. middle-aged people

33. Mr. Jones, age 85, has a terminal diagnosis of lung cancer. His primary source of payment for home care services would most likely be:

    A. private health insurance

    B. worker's compensation

    C. HMO

    D. Medicare hospice

34. The patient has been discharged from a hospital to his or her environment and requires daily nursing care. Who will provide the care?

    A. long-term care

    B. home health care

    C. subacute care

    D. skilled nursing facility

35. The health care team member who coordinates community resources to meet patient and/or family needs is the:
    A. LPN
    B. RN
    C. public health nurse
    D. social worker

36. All of the following are functions of the home care aide except:
    A. bathing the patient
    B. reporting problems
    C. documentation
    D. inserting an indwelling (Foley) catheter

37. Which condition should the home care aide report to the nurse supervisor?
    A. open reddened area
    B. cooperative patient
    C. normal bowel habits
    D. amount eaten for lunch

38. Which statement should the home care aide understand regarding observation of patients?
    A. Only licensed nurses do observation.
    B. Abnormal observations are not reported.
    C. Observation is not a continuous process.
    D. Observation begins the first time you see the patient.

39. The home care aide must report abnormal observations to which health care team member?
    A. nurse supervisor
    B. agency administrator
    C. physician
    D. family member

40. Which of the following is *not* part of the home care aide's dress code?
    A. uniform according to agency policy
    B. loose, dangling earrings
    C. identification badge
    D. nails short and clean

41. All of the following are forms of body language communication except:
    A. facial expressions
    B. gestures
    C. touch
    D. speech

42. An example of a patient with a sensory impairment is one who is:
    A. obese
    B. hyperactive
    C. blind
    D. bed-bound

43. Your patient's daughter arrives at the house and tells you, "While I'm here to watch Mama, you clean the bathroom." What is your appropriate response?
    A. "I don't clean bathrooms."
    B. "My supervisor sets up the plan of care. I must discuss all changes with her."
    C. "Sure, I'm glad to help."
    D. "Honey, I don't even clean my own bathroom!"

44. All of the following are examples of tact except:
    A. answering the patient's question promptly
    B. showing frustration each time the patient calls for help
    C. being considerate at all times
    D. encouraging the patient to do as much for himself or herself as possible

45. Exposing a patient's body unnecessarily is an example of:
    A. criminal law
    B. libel
    C. invasion of privacy
    D. battery

46. Which of the following actions by the home care aide would demonstrate confidentiality?
    A. discussing the patient's health status with neighbors
    B. talking about the patient with coworkers who are not on the case
    C. discussing the patient's concerns with the nurse supervisor
    D. discussing the patient's health status with the patient's pastor

47. An objective observation is all of the following except:
    A. what the home care aide can see
    B. what the patient states
    C. what the home care aide can feel
    D. what the home care aide can hear

48. An example of a subjective observation is:
    A. headache
    B. red eyes
    C. rash
    D. edema

49. Teaching patients is an important part of your job. You will teach patients by:
    A. example
    B. discussion
    C. taking part in patient activities
    D. all of the above

50. One of your coworkers shared her marital problems with one of your patients, who then shared this information with you. This situation has challenged your:
    A. code of ethics
    B. senses
    C. thinking
    D. stamina

51. As a home care aide, you will be able to:
    A. give basic care in an emergency
    B. perform sterile dressing changes

C. insert an indwelling (Foley) catheter
D. change IV sites

52. You come to work every day, and you come on time. Your supervisor can rely on you to do things at the proper time and in the proper way. This describes the home care aide quality of:
    A. accuracy
    B. following directions
    C. dependability
    D. cleanliness

53. All of the following are forms of written communication except:
    A. a drawing
    B. instructions left in the home by the nurse
    C. a note describing your activities with a patient
    D. a voice mail message

54. Your supervisor tells you about an assignment. This is a form of:
    A. written communication
    B. verbal communication
    C. nonverbal communication
    D. body language

55. The patient refuses personal care. Which one of the following should the home care aide do?
    A. force the patient to receive personal care
    B. ignore the patient
    C. report the problem to the nurse supervisor
    D. leave the patient's home immediately

56. Calling your patient "honey" or "sugar" is a violation of which of the patient's rights?
    A. the right to civil and religious liberties
    B. the right to be treated with respect
    C. the right to privacy
    D. the right to refuse care

57. Your patient is confined to bed in his bedroom. What is an appropriate way for him to signal for your help?

A. a hand bell

B. a stick used to bang on the bed or floor

C. a voice signal

D. all of the above

58. Upon arrival at your patient's home, you hear the patient's wife and daughter arguing about what the patient should eat for breakfast. The daughter asks you what you think. What is the appropriate response?

A. "Your idea is fine."

B. "Mrs. Smith knows what's best for her husband."

C. "I really think you should settle this between yourselves."

D. "I don't care. Feed him whatever you want."

59. You observe a skin rash and swelling of the patient's feet. You are using which sense for your observations?

A. sight

B. touch

C. hearing

D. smell

60. You notice that your patient's skin is cool, moist, and bumpy. You are using which sense for your observations?

A. sight

B. touch

C. hearing

D. smell

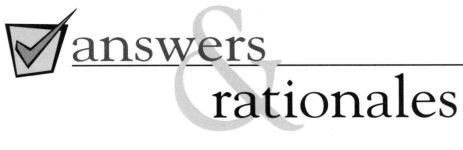
answers & rationales

1.

C. The goal of the home health team is to provide care so that the patient can function optimally and administrators are not involved in direct care. *(Zucker, p. 7)*

2.

B. A judgmental attitude is *not* needed by home care aides. *(Zucker, p. 20)*

3.

A. The tasks and responsibilities expected of you are summarized in your job description. *(Zucker, p. 8)*

4.

B. This is the description of responsibilities for the physical therapist. *(Zucker, p. 7)*

5.

D. ALL of the qualities are part of the most effective qualities to succeed as a home care aide. *(Zucker, p. 11)*

6.

C. Your supervisor will help you to learn and understand your job. *(Zucker, p. 8)*

7.

A. Your agency has a protocol (set of plans or procedures) for deciding the method of payment that patients will use. If patients have questions, refer them to your supervisor. *(Zucker, pp. 6–7)*

8.

D. Teamwork means that everyone knows what she or he is supposed to do. *(Zucker, p. 8)*

9.

C. Dependability means that your supervisor can rely on you to do things at the proper time and in the proper way. *(Zucker, p. 11)*

10.

A. There is a reason for every step of the patient's care, so you must be very careful and accurate in caring for patients. *(Zucker, p. 11)*

11.

C. Home care aides will work within an accepted set of rules of moral behavior and beliefs. Ethics is a code of rules set up to govern behavior. *(Zucker, p. 12)*

12.

D. Confidentiality is an important part of patient care. *(Zucker, p. 12)*

13.

B. Negligence is a legal term meaning the failure to give proper care when you know how to do so. *(Zucker, p. 13)*

14.

B. An incident is an event that does not fit the daily routine of the home or agency where you are working. *(Zucker, p. 13)*

15.

A. Your supervisor is the person directly responsible for your activities. *(Zucker, p. 13)*

16.

A. Speaking is a form of verbal communication. *(Zucker, p. 18)*

17.

C. Body language is a nonverbal way in which gestures function as a form of communication. *(Zucker, p. 18)*

18.

C. Body language gives silent clues to others about how you feel and what you want other people to do. Speaking is not silent! *(Zucker, p. 18)*

19.

D. Home care aides must be courteous, tactful, and sensitive in communicating with people. *(Zucker, pp. 20–21)*

20.

D. Breathing changes, bleeding, and pain are all changes in patient condition that must be reported. *(Zucker, p. 24)*

21.

B. You are the health care team member who will spend the most time with the patient, so your observations are very important. *(Zucker, p. 23)*

22.

B. If the home care aide has a concern about something that happens with the patient, this information should be reported to the supervisor only. *(Zucker, p. 23)*

23.

C. The appropriate practice is to document care as soon as possible after it is provided. *(Zucker, p. 26)*

24.

A. Subjective reporting is giving your opinion about what you have observed. This may be very important to the care of your patient. B and C are examples of objective reporting. *(Zucker, p. 24)*

25.

B. Subjective reporting is giving your opinion about what you have observed. This may be very important to the care of your patient. *(Zucker, p. 24)*

26.

A. This statement is an opinion and an example of subjective reporting. *(Zucker, p. 24)*

27.

D. Reporting all changes in a patient's condition and reporting events in the order in which they occur are two of the basic guidelines for reporting and recording. *(Zucker, p. 27)*

28.

B. Every patient has the right to be able to participate in his or her plan of care. *(Zucker, p. 5)*

29.

A. Confidentiality is a very important part of patient care and permits you to discuss patient information with your supervisor. *(Zucker, p. 12)*

30.

D. This is NOT included in the patient's bill of rights. *(Zucker, p. 5)*

31.

A. This IS the primary function of the home care aide. *(Zucker, p. 7)*

32.

B. The elderly and low-income individuals benefit from Medicare and Medicaid. *(Zucker, p. 6)*

33.

D. Mr. Jones fits the eligibility criteria for Medicare Hospice. *(Zucker, p. 6)*

34.

B. Home health care is provided to patients in their homes—their own environments—not in the other facilities listed. *(Zucker, p. 2)*

35.

D. This is part of the formal training and role of the social worker, not of the nursing staff. *(Zucker, p. 7)*

36.

D. A, B, and C are functions of the home care aide. D is the function of a skilled professional. *(Zucker, p. 9)*

37.

A. An open reddened area is an observation of something that is not normal, and it should be reported. *(Zucker, p. 23)*

38.

D. Observation absolutely begins the first time you see the patient and is continuous and may be performed by any member of the health care team. *(Zucker, p. 23)*

39.

A. It is an important part of the home care aide's job to report changes to the nurse supervisor, who will then take appropriate actions. *(Zucker, p. 23)*

40.

B. Do not wear jewelry such as earrings, bracelets, pendants, or large rings while providing care on the job. The other items will be part of the dress code. *(Zucker, p. 14)*

41.

D. Speech is a form of verbal communication, while facial expressions, gestures, and touch are forms of body language communication. *(Zucker, p. 18)*

42.

C. Blindness is an impairment of the sense of sight. *(Zucker, p. 23)*

43.

B. Be open about your responsibilities. Explaining that your supervisor sets up the plan of care and makes changes is open and responsible. *(Zucker, p. 22)*

44.

B. Tact means doing and saying the right thing at the right time. *(Zucker, p. 21)*

45.

C. An important patient right is the right to privacy. *(Zucker, p. 5)*

46.

C. You should discuss patient-related issues only with people who are directly involved with the patient's care, such as your nurse supervisor. *(Zucker, p. 12)*

47.

B. What the patient states is an example of a subjective observation. *(Zucker, p. 24)*

48.

A. Subjective observations are signs and symptoms that can be felt and described only by the patient. *(Zucker, p. 24)*

49.

D. These teaching methods will help you teach new skills, relearn old skills, and help the patient gain independence. *(Zucker, p. 28)*

50.

A. It is assumed that home care aides work within an accepted set of rules—ethics—and that they do not discuss personal problems with patients. *(Zucker, p. 12)*

51.

A. Of the skills listed, the only one within the scope of practice of the home care aide is giving basic care in an emergency. Skilled professionals perform the remaining skills. *(Zucker, p. 9)*

52.

C. This is an exact description of dependability as a home care aide. *(Zucker, p. 11)*

53.

D. Anything you communicate through writing is written communication. A voice mail message is verbal communication. *(Zucker, p. 18)*

54.

B. Verbal communication is the exchange of ideas or information through the spoken word. *(Zucker, p. 18)*

55.

C. Home care patients have the right to refuse care. Report this to your supervisor. *(Zucker, p. 5)*

56.

B. Patients have the right to be treated with respect, and this includes addressing them by their desired names and/or titles. *(Zucker, p. 5)*

57.

D. Every patient needs a way to signal to other people. Use whatever method is most appropriate in the house where you are working. *(Zucker, p. 19)*

58.

C. Try not to get involved in family affairs. Never take sides in a family quarrel. *(Zucker, p. 22)*

59.

A. You can see some signs of change in a patient's condition, such as using your eyes to observe a rash and swelling of the feet. *(Zucker, p. 23)*

60.

B. You can feel some changes in the patient's conditions with your hands, such as skin temperature, moisture, and texture. *(Zucker, p. 23)*

2 Patient Populations

chapter objectives

Upon completion of Chapter 2, the student is responsible for the following:

➤ Describe geriatrics.

➤ Identify common disease processes and their effects on the body.

➤ Identify the role of the home care aide in caring for patients with common diseases.

➤ Describe dressing techniques.

➤ Describe care of infants and children.

DIRECTIONS
Each of the questions or incomplete statements below is followed by four suggested answers or completions. Select **one answer** that is best in each case.

1. The AIDS infection may affect:
   A. any segment of the population
   B. only homosexual populations
   C. only bisexual and homosexual populations
   D. only people who have weakened immune systems

2. Symptoms of AIDS include:
   A. weakness
   B. debilitation
   C. difficulty breathing
   D. all of the above

3. Which of the following should you avoid when preparing meals for the patient with AIDS?
   A. candy
   B. carbohydrates
   C. raw eggs and raw meat
   D. sugar

4. Patients with AIDS are at medical risk for:
   A. numerous infections
   B. loss of job
   C. depression
   D. A and C

5. Symptoms experienced by many patients suffering from AIDS include:
   A. vomiting
   B. diarrhea
   C. poor appetite
   D. all of the above

6. Alzheimer's disease is characterized by:
   A. confusion
   B. restlessness
   C. increased independence
   D. A and B

7. A safety consideration for the patient with Alzheimer's disease includes:
   A. wandering
   B. restlessness
   C. incontinence
   D. fear of food

8. An important consideration in caring for the patient with an amputation is:
   A. completing patient's activities for him/her
   B. encouraging patient not to talk about the amputation
   C. helping the patient achieve and maintain balance
   D. none of the above

9. It is extremely important in caring for the patient with arthritis that:
   A. the home care aide provide all care
   B. affected joints be immobilized
   C. joints be maintained in functional positions
   D. none of the above

10. Symptoms of a brain tumor may include:
    A. headache
    B. vomiting
    C. seizures
    D. all of the above

11. When a patient is experiencing a seizure, the home care aide should:
    A. try to restrain the patient
    B. put a metal spoon in the patient's mouth
    C. protect the patient from hurting himself or herself
    D. immediately call the patient's physician

12. To provide security and consistency in caring for the patient with Alzheimer's disease, it is important to provide:
    A. sweets
    B. strict routine
    C. discipline
    D. frequent naps

13. An 85-year-old female patient had a right mastectomy 20 years ago. In taking her blood pressure, it is important to remember:
    A. that 160/90 would be a normal reading
    B. that she will have lower blood pressure if she is in bed
    C. to take the blood pressure in her right arm
    D. to take blood pressure in her leg

14. When caring for a patient who is undergoing radiation therapy, you should NOT:
    A. give a bed bath
    B. wash off the skin markings
    C. give a shampoo
    D. assist with dressing

15. Patients who have osteoporosis may have weakened bones and are at greater risk for:
    A. pathological fractures
    B. arthritis
    C. fatigue
    D. infection

16. Patients who have cancer and are undergoing chemotherapy should be encouraged to:
    A. take long walks to increase strength
    B. eat nutritious meals and snacks
    C. eat very little
    D. brush their gums vigorously

17. If your patient has chronic heart disease, it is important to remember:
    A. that long walks increase strength
    B. that deep breathing exercises increase endurance
    C. that frequent rest periods are necessary during care
    D. to give heart medicine before you leave

18. Which of the following is not a sign or symptom of a heart attack?
    A. pink color
    B. weak pulse
    C. chest pain
    D. wet, clammy skin

19. Mr. Tucker has swelling in his right ankle. You know that he has chronic heart disease. You should encourage him to:
    A. remain in bed as much as possible
    B. elevate his foot as much as possible
    C. avoid walking and use a wheelchair
    D. drink lots of water

20. When considering the condition of a patient with heart disease, it is important to report which of the following?
    A. quiet respirations
    B. pink nailbeds
    C. blue color of lips, fingers, and toes
    D. warm skin

21. While caring for your patient with angina, she complains of shortness of breath. You should
    A. call an ambulance
    B. turn up the oxygen setting
    C. allow her to rest
    D. complete the bath and then allow her to rest

22. Common effects of stroke include:
    A. paralysis on the affected side
    B. steady gait
    C. good balance
    D. clear speech

23. Your patient has had a stroke and has difficulty swallowing. After you assist him with feeding, he should be positioned:

    A. on his side

    B. on his back

    C. flat in bed

    D. with his head tilted forward

24. Cerebrovascular accidents (CVA) may be caused by:

    A. blood clot in the leg

    B. blood clot in the arm

    C. blood clot in the brain

    D. blood clot in the lungs

25. Therapists who may be involved with the care of the patient recovering from a CVA include:

    A. physical therapists

    B. occupational therapists

    C. speech therapists

    D. all of the above

26. When caring for a patient with left-sided weakness, the home care aide should:

    A. perform all ADLs for the patient

    B. change the patient's schedule

    C. assist the patient to dress the left side first

    D. place food on the patient's left side

27. You are visiting an 8-year-old child. Her primary caregiver will most likely be:

    A. her uncle

    B. her mother

    C. the social worker

    D. siblings

28. Chronic obstructive pulmonary disease (COPD) includes diseases such as:

    A. emphysema

    B. cancer

    C. acute bronchitis

    D. flu

29. Patients with COPD frequently receive oxygen. While providing personal care, it is important to:

    A. give the bath without any breaks

    B. perform all ADLs for these patients

    C. give only bed baths

    D. remove or turn off the oxygen when using a blow dryer

30. Patients with COPD have a high level of carbon dioxide building up in their systems. This may result in:

    A. unusual behavior and not being able to be left alone

    B. fruity breath

    C. pink skin

    D. constipation

31. Diabetes mellitus is a disease in which the body is unable to:

    A. break down protein

    B. break down fat

    C. break down carbohydrates

    D. break down vitamins

32. Foot care for the diabetic patient may include:

    A. cutting the toenails

    B. scrubbing the heels with a brush

    C. drying between the patient's toes

    D. applying powder

33. Symptoms of low blood sugar (hypoglycemia) include:

    A. excessive urine

    B. extreme thirst

    C. feeling nervous and irritable

    D. increased activity

34. Symptoms of high blood sugar (hyperglycemia) include:

    A. perspiration

    B. feeling jittery

C. increased urination

D. hunger

35. The bones of an elderly person are:

A. stronger than those of a younger person

B. denser than those of a younger person

C. the same size as those of a younger person

D. more brittle than those of a younger person

36. Assisting the patient with diabetes with his or her care involves all of the following except:

A. giving the patient insulin injections

B. testing the urine for sugar and acetone

C. foot care

D. lubricating the skin

37. Patients with Parkinson's disease may experience symptoms such as:

A. tremors of hands or legs

B. difficulty walking

C. slowness of movement

D. all of the above

38. When caring for a patient who is confused or mentally ill, you should remember to:

A. talk about your family

B. talk about the daily news

C. talk about familiar objects, people, and events

D. talk about the other caregivers

39. A patient with osteoarthritis complains of feeling stiff and difficulty moving. You can assist by:

A. encouraging fluids

B. applying ice packs

C. giving a warm bath or shower if a part of her treatment plan

D. asking the nurse to give more medications

40. You are caring for a patient with osteoporosis. When providing care, it is important to remember to:

A. use very hot water for bathing

B. provide for safety

C. apply adult briefs

D. lift the patient into the tub

41. Your patient is recovering from a stroke. He hesitates when trying to dress himself. How can the home care aide help?

A. Tell him to do another task.

B. Finish dressing him.

C. Leave him in pajamas.

D. Remind him what to do next.

42. Miss Darby has had a severe stroke and is unconscious. In providing care for her, you should always:

A. talk to her and tell her what you are doing

B. turn on the radio and listen to your favorite music

C. whisper

D. talk to the family about television shows

43. When helping your patient select clothing to wear, which of the following would you not consider?

A. the patient's physical capabilities

B. the patient's preferences

C. your personal preferences

D. changing weather conditions

44. Keeping furniture and belongings in the same place is very important for elderly patients with:

A. hearing loss

B. bone disease

C. visual impairments

D. heart disease

45. Stage I of Alzheimer's disease is characterized by:

A. lack of speech

B. confinement to bed

C. refusal to eat

D. covering up of memory loss

46. Stage II of Alzheimer's disease is characterized by:
    A. wandering
    B. repetitive movements
    C. continual pacing in small areas
    D. all of the above

47. Stage III of Alzheimer's disease is characterized by:
    A. unresponsiveness
    B. pacing
    C. wandering
    D. increased talking

48. Mr. White has had Alzheimer's disease for nine years and has been cared for at home by his family and other caregivers. You notice some family tension. You should:
    A. tell them to get counseling
    B. report this to your supervisor
    C. ignore the tension
    D. tell them about your weekend activities

49. The spread of cancer cells from one area to another is called:
    A. metastasis
    B. malignant
    C. benign
    D. biopsy

50. As hypertension develops, people may complain of:
    A. headaches
    B. hearing changes
    C. incontinence
    D. all of the above

51. You have a higher risk of hypertension if you:
    A. smoke cigarettes
    B. are white
    C. eat a diet high in carbohydrates
    D. exercise

52. Your patient has hypertension and is taking medications to control it. She develops a cold and begins to take some over-the-counter medications on her own. You should:
    A. encourage her to take the new medications regularly
    B. assist her with taking the new medications
    C. report the new medications to your supervisor
    D. call her doctor

53. Death of a part of the heart due to a blockage in a blood vessel is known as:
    A. hypertension
    B. myocardial infarction
    C. cerebrovascular accident
    D. angina

54. In caring for a patient with a pacemaker, you must remember to:
    A. report when your patient has hiccups
    B. report incontinence
    C. report constipation
    D. encourage high fluid intake

55. The purpose of a pacemaker is to:
    A. increase urinary output
    B. relieve constipation
    C. regulate the heart rhythm
    D. cure hypertension

56. In caring for the elderly, the home care aide should realize that aging affects:
    A. circulation
    B. skin
    C. mobility
    D. all of the above

57. Why might an older person need to urinate more frequently than a younger person does?
    A. An older person needs to drink more fluids
    B. Older people like to spend time in the bathroom
    C. The bladder of an older person is smaller in size
    D. Older people are generally confused

58. Patients with Alzheimer's disease must be:
    A. restrained
    B. told what to do just like children
    C. supervised closely but not restrained
    D. sent to nursing homes

59. When meeting a child as a patient:
    A. talk only to the parents
    B. bend down so that you are at eye level
    C. tell the child that you are there to take over for his or her mother
    D. all of the above

60. Reasons why a home care aide may care for a child include which of the following?
    A. The primary caregiver becomes ill or disabled.
    B. The primary caregiver must be taught, by example, how to care for the child.
    C. Child abuse or neglect has been reported or suspected.
    D. all of the above

61. In caring for children, the home care aide should consider:
    A. treating them as little adults
    B. that their basic needs are less than those of adults
    C. that their reactions and needs are based on their experiences as children
    D. focusing attention on the parents

62. While caring for a 36-year-old woman who has a new colostomy, you should remember that her 8-month-old daughter's primary activities are:
    A. toilet training
    B. learning to walk
    C. routines of eating, sleeping, and simple play
    D. all of the above

63. Your patient is a 15-year-old paraplegic. Key characteristics of adolescence include:
    A. mood changes

B. attachment to mother
    C. lack of modesty
    D. dependence

64. Congenital anomalies are known as:
    A. injuries
    B. birth defects
    C. punishments
    D. developmental characteristics

65. Birth defects may result from:
    A. only genetic disorders
    B. drug or alcohol abuse during pregnancy
    C. a high-fat diet during pregnancy
    D. normal activities

66. The family of a child with a congenital anomaly may experience:
    A. anger
    B. guilt
    C. emotional difficulties
    D. all of the above

67. Children who are ill may react to their illnesses by:
    A. playing more
    B. nightmares and fears
    C. passive behaviors
    D. doing more chores

68. A set of rules that govern conduct and actions resulting in orderly behavior is known as:
    A. punishment
    B. discipline
    C. ethics
    D. laws

69. An action performed as the result of wrongdoing is known as:
    A. discipline
    B. penance
    C. punishment
    D. abuse

70. The child in your care throws a glass and breaks it. You should:
    A. spank the child
    B. tell the child that you love him, but you don't like what he did, and remove an activity
    C. make the child clean up the glass
    D. lock the child in his room

71. Appropriate responses to children's behavior include all of the following except:
    A. "I expect you to eat your cereal. Do you understand?"
    B. "You're going to get in big trouble for this."
    C. "Please lower the TV because it is disturbing your Grandpa, and he can't sleep."
    D. "You may play outside until dark and then come in. Do you understand?"

72. Any act that causes another person harm is:
    A. abuse
    B. punishment
    C. discipline
    D. neglect

73. All of the following are some reasons for child abuse except that:
    A. the abuser was also abused as a child
    B. the abuser has normal mental health
    C. the abuser cannot cope with the stress of having a child
    D. the abuser is not the parent, but the parent is unable to stop the event

74. Children may not report abuse because:
    A. they are ashamed
    B. they are afraid the abuse will increase
    C. they feel they deserve it
    D. all of the above

75. Forms of child abuse include all of the following except:
    A. physical
    B. financial
    C. emotional
    D. sexual

76. There are small children who live in the home where you care for a 68-year-old woman. You unexpectedly notice small circular burn marks on the arm of a 2-year-old girl. You should:
    A. apply first aid cream to the burns
    B. notify your supervisor immediately
    C. ask all the children what happened
    D. put bandages on the marks

77. Home care aides may care for infants in the home because:
    A. the mother is recovering from surgery
    B. the infant is being abused
    C. there are many other children in the house
    D. all of the above

78. The most important part of your role when caring for an infant is:
    A. baths
    B. teaching by example
    C. feeding
    D. diaper changes

79. Most infants are fed:
    A. every 1 to 2 hours
    B. every 3 to 4 hours
    C. every 5 to 6 hours
    D. every 7 to 8 hours

80. Factors to consider when carrying an infant include all except which of the following?
    A. Always support the child's head.
    B. Talking on the phone while holding an infant is permissible.
    C. Hold the infant close to you.
    D. Be alert while carrying a baby up and down stairs.

81. Special considerations for the nursing mother include all except which of the following?

A. The mother should eat a balanced diet.

B. The mother should drink 6 to 8 glasses of fluid each day.

C. The mother should decrease her calorie intake to lose weight.

D. The mother should take vitamins if the physician recommends them.

82. Guidelines for the home care aide to assist with bottle-feeding include all except which of the following?

    A. Prop the bottle up on a pillow while the baby is lying in the crib.

    B. Always check the temperature of the liquid before giving it to the baby.

    C. Make sure the formula is fresh and the bottles have been properly stored.

    D. The nipple should be full of liquid to prevent the baby from sucking and swallowing air.

83. The home care aide is asked to sterilize baby bottles and nipples. The most common method is:

    A. in the dishwasher

    B. on the top of the stove

    C. in the microwave

    D. in an autoclave

84. When sterilizing baby bottles on top of the stove in boiling water, allow the water to boil for:

    A. 10 minutes

    B. 15 minutes

    C. 20 minutes

    D. 25 minutes

85. The least expensive type of infant formula is:

    A. concentrated liquid formula

    B. powdered formula

    C. prepared formula

    D. natural formula

86. Infant formula may be refrigerated for how long without spoiling?

    A. 12 hours

    B. 24 hours

    C. 2 days

    D. 3 days

87. Guidelines for changing infant diapers include all except which of the following?

    A. Change the diapers often to decrease odor and skin irritation.

    B. Use rubber pants over disposable diapers.

    C. Clean the baby's genital area each time you change the diaper.

    D. Do not flush disposable diapers down a toilet.

88. Guidelines for care of an infant's umbilical cord include all except which of the following?

    A. Pull off a dried and scabby cord after 10 days.

    B. Keep the diaper folded down away from the cord.

    C. Wash the umbilical cord with plain rubbing alcohol at every diaper change.

    D. Never give the infant a tub bath until the cord falls off.

89. Guidelines for care of a baby boy's circumcision include:

    A. bleeding is expected for 10 days

    B. drainage is expected for 10 days

    C. keep the penis clean and free of fecal matter

    D. give him a bath every diaper change

90. Your patient has a lower leg cast from a broken ankle. You should report to your supervisor:

    A. that the patient wiggles his toes

    B. that the patient's skin is pink above the cast

    C. unusual odors coming from the cast

    D. that the patient's toes are ticklish

91. Guidelines for caring for a patient with a cast include all except which of the following?
    A. Pain is normal when wearing a cast.
    B. Casts should not restrict circulation.
    C. Do not put anything into the cast.
    D. Do not get the cast wet.

92. The joints that are most commonly affected by arthritis include all of the following except the:
    A. shoulders
    B. ankles
    C. jaw
    D. fingers

93. Your elderly patient has joint pain in her knees every time she moves. She complains that it feels as though the bones are rubbing against each other. You note that her right knee is red and swollen. She has a type of arthritis that is common among the elderly known as:
    A. osteoarthritis
    B. rheumatoid arthritis
    C. gout
    D. ankylosing spondylitis

94. Mr. Taylor is a 71-year-old man with Parkinson's disease. Which of the following should be reported to your supervisor?
    A. hand tremors
    B. he stopped taking his medications
    C. slow gait
    D. drooling

95. Mrs. Kyle is a 32-year-old woman with multiple sclerosis (MS). Which of the following should be reported to your supervisor?
    A. She tires easily.
    B. Her 8-year-old son has chicken pox.
    C. She cries when watching TV.
    D. Sometimes her speech is not clear.

96. Guidelines for caring for a patient with amyotrophic lateral sclerosis (ALS) include all except which of the following?
    A. Medications must be taken as scheduled.
    B. Encourage the patient to be as independent as possible.
    C. Eat small meals high in nutrients and fiber.
    D. Change the exercise routine.

97. Acquired immune deficiency syndrome (AIDS) is best described as the body's inability to:
    A. digest food
    B. eliminate waste
    C. fight infections
    D. circulate blood

98. You can teach your patient ways to decrease the spread of tuberculosis (TB). This includes all except which of the following?
    A. The patient must wear a mask.
    B. Coughing or sneezing into a tissue.
    C. Wash hands frequently.
    D. Do not touch hands to eyes, nose, or mouth.

99. Symptoms of tuberculosis include all of the following except:
    A. coughing up blood
    B. weight gain
    C. fever
    D. sweating, especially at night

100. The family members of a patient with TB are worried about catching the disease. Inform them:
    A. to isolate the patient
    B. that once TB is under treatment, the chance of catching TB is past
    C. to wash all of the patient's dishes separately
    D. to wash all of the patient's linens separately

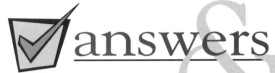
answers & rationales

1.

A. AIDS is spread as a virus through sexual contact between two people and by sharing IV drug equipment when one person is infected with the virus. *(Zucker, pp. 372–373)*

2.

C. Often AIDS patients have difficulty breathing, so be alert to possible changes in their ability to breathe or speak. *(Zucker, p. 373)*

3.

C. The patient with AIDS has a compromised immune system and is unable to tolerate raw foods of animal origin. *(Model Curriculum, p. 323)*

4.

D. Their immune system is compromised, and they are at risk for infections. They are at risk for depression because of the huge impact that AIDS has on their lives. *(Model Curriculum, pp. 323–324)*

5.

D. This is due to the changes in their immune systems. *(Model Curriculum, p. 323)*

6.

D. Alzheimer's disease is the major cause of mental deterioration among people over the age of 65. *(Zucker, p. 365)*

7.

A. Be alert for the safety of the patient. *(Zucker, p. 365)*

8.

C. Rehabilitation is the process of relearning how to function and in the best possible and most safe way. *(Zucker, p. 233)*

9.

C. Arthritis is a chronic disease. It is important to keep joints functioning in the best possible way. *(Zucker, pp. 233, 362)*

10.

D. When part of the brain is damaged or invaded by a tumor, the path along which nerve impulses travel is damaged, and the patient may have these symptoms. *(Zucker, p. 102)*

11.

C. Your role in caring for a patient having a seizure is to prevent the patient from injuring himself or herself. *(Zucker, p. 341)*

12.

B. Follow the care plan carefully. The maintenance of a routine is one way to ease the care of the patient. *(Zucker, p. 365)*

13.

B. A person's circulation tends to slow down when she is in bed. *(Zucker, p. 104)*

14.

B. These skin markings are drawn to indicate the target for radiation. Do not wash off the marks. *(Zucker, p. 200)*

15.

A. As we age, our bones become more brittle. Elderly patients are at risk for osteoporosis, which is weakening of the bone, placing them at risk for pathological fractures. *(Zucker, p. 100)*

16.

B. Many people who are receiving chemotherapy and radiation therapy change their eating habits because of periods of nausea, vomiting, appetite loss, and/or constipation. Encourage them to eat small, frequent meals. *(Zucker, p. 172)*

17.

C. Balance activity and rest with these patients. Discuss changes with your supervisor. *(Zucker, p. 354)*

18.

A. The skin will be pale in color. *(Zucker, p. 353)*

19.

B. If an arm or leg is swollen, try to keep the part higher than the heart. Gravity will help the extra fluid to drain from the limb. *(Zucker, p. 183)*

20.

C. A blue or gray color of the lips, nails, fingers, or toes is indication of a lack of circulating oxygen. *(Zucker, p. 24)*

21.

C. Usually, the discomfort disappears after resting and medication. *(Zucker, p. 355)*

22.

A. The results of a CVA may be paralysis and loss of speech or vision. *(Zucker, p. 359)*

23.

A. Turning the patient onto her side reduces the risk of aspiration. *(Zucker, p. 107)*

24.

C. A CVA occurs when the blood supply to a part of the brain is stopped because of a blocked blood vessel. *(Zucker, p. 360)*

25.

D. These therapists will plan an individualized program for your patient. *(Zucker, p. 361)*

26.

C. The involved or affected side is first into the garment and last out. *(Zucker, p. 207)*

27.

B. The main caregiver is usually a parent. *(Zucker, p. 61)*

28.

A. COPD refers to diseases that cause permanent damage to lung tissue, including emphysema, asthma, and chronic bronchitis. *(Zucker, p. 366)*

29.

D. Do not use electrical appliances such as heating pads, hair dryers, or electric shavers near oxygen. *(Zucker, p. 154)*

30.

A. Their lungs are not able to eliminate waste products, such as carbon dioxide, and they may exhibit unusual behaviors and may be unable to make decisions or be left alone. *(Zucker, p. 366)*

31.

C. Diabetes is a condition in which the body cannot change carbohydrates into energy because of an imbalance of insulin. *(Zucker, p. 357)*

32.

C. Many diabetics have difficulty with their feet. Be sure to dry between the toes before putting on socks or footwear. *(Zucker, p. 359)*

33.

C. Irritability, personality changes, and nervousness are symptoms of hypoglycemia. The other choices are symptoms of hyperglycemia. *(Zucker, p. 358)*

34.

C. Excessive urination is a symptom of hyperglycemia. The other choices are symptoms of hypoglycemia. *(Zucker, p. 358)*

35.

D. As we age, our bones become more brittle. Fractures mend slowly. *(Zucker, p. 100)*

36.

A. You may assist your patient with medication, but never give an injection or oral medication. *(Zucker, p. 358)*

37.

D. These and other symptoms—changes in vision, drooling, difficulty swallowing, and bowel and bladder incontinence—are experienced. *(Zucker, p. 368)*

38.

C. The familiar and the routine will enhance care of the patient. *(Zucker, p. 365)*

39.

C. If it's a part of her treatment plan wet heat may be very soothing and helpful to stiff, painful joints. *(Zucker, p. 362)*

40.

B. Safety is essential for these patients with extremely brittle bones. *(Zucker, p. 100)*

41.

D. Reminding and encouraging the patient helps him to complete the task. *(Zucker, pp. 264–265)*

42.

A. Even though the patient may be unconscious, she may still be able to hear you. *(Zucker, p. 206)*

43.

C. Let the patient select what he would like to wear and do as much of the actual dressing as possible. *(Zucker, p. 264)*

44.

C. For the elderly, poor eyesight, decreased reflexes, and poor hearing all contribute to accidents. Don't move things! *(Zucker, p. 55)*

45.

D. In the beginning stage, patients are able to cover up memory loss, decreased speech, and even emotional agitation, depression, or apathy. *(Zucker, p. 365)*

46.

D. During this period, which may extend over many years, the patient's memory progressively worsens, and behaviors may seem very meaningless and repetitive. *(Zucker, p. 365)*

47.

A. This is the terminal stage, and the patient may become unresponsive. *(Zucker, p. 366)*

48.

B. Be alert to family tension, and report this to your supervisor, who will discuss appropriate counseling or support groups. *(Zucker, p. 366)*

49.

A. This is the definition of metastasis. *(Zucker, p. 364)*

50.

A. As hypertension develops, people may complain of headaches, vision changes, or problems with urinary output. *(Zucker, p. 351)*

51.

A. Smoking cigarettes is a significant factor in risk for hypertension. *(Zucker, p. 35)*

52.

C. If your patient starts taking any medications, including nonprescription drugs, report this to your supervisor. *(Zucker, p. 352)*

53.

B. Myocardial infarction (MI) is also known as a heart attack and is death of heart tissue due to blockage in a blood vessel. *(Zucker, p. 352)*

54.

A. Hiccups should be reported immediately, as this could be an indication that the electrical wires are out of place. *(Zucker, p. 355)*

55.

C. A pacemaker is an electrical device used to stimulate the heart and regulate the rhythm. *(Zucker, p. 354)*

56.

D. Aging affects all body systems. Some experience more changes as a result of aging than others. *(Zucker, p. 54)*

57.

C. A normal change of aging is a decrease in the size of the urinary bladder, resulting in frequency of urination. *(Zucker, p. 55)*

58.

C. The brain cannot process familiar information, and the patient is not able to function. These patients need very close supervision, routines, and regularly scheduled activities. *(Zucker, p. 365)*

59.

B. Get at eye level with the child and spend a few minutes alone with the child. This will let him or her know that he or she is important and allow both of you to get to know each other. *(Zucker, p. 66)*

60.

D. In addition, the primary caregiver may need rest or assistance with the care of the child with an illness or disability or must leave the house to work. *(Zucker, p. 66)*

61.

C. Children have the same physical and emotional needs as adults. They depend on adults to meet their needs. They are not little adults, and their reactions and needs are based on their experiences as children. *(Zucker, p. 66)*

62.

C. Infants experience rapid growth and are totally dependent on adults. Provide calm routines, taking into account the infant's schedule. *(Zucker, p. 68)*

63.

A. This is a period of rapid physical and emotional changes, including mood swings. Independence and privacy are very important. *(Zucker, p. 68)*

64.

B. Congenital anomalies are deviations from the normal features that are present at birth and are known as birth defects. *(Zucker, p. 67)*

65.

B. Birth defects may result from genetic disorder or from external factors, such as exposure to toxic substances, drug use, or alcohol abuse during pregnancy. *(Zucker, p. 67)*

66.

D. It is not unusual for the family to experience anger, guilt, denial, and emotional difficulties as they learn to care for this child. *(Zucker, p. 67)*

67.

B. Children may behave in a manner that is unusual, offensive, and difficult to explain. You may notice shyness and withdrawal, nightmares and fears, aggressive behaviors, and refusal to follow familiar routines, among other unusual behaviors. *(Zucker, p. 69)*

68.

B. Discipline is a system of rules, which may be well known. *(Zucker, p. 69)*

69.

C. Punishment is a harsh act given as a result of an offense or wrongdoing, as when a rule or discipline is broken. *(Zucker, p. 69)*

70.

B. Your role is to maintain the discipline already in the home. Punishment is not within your role in the home. *(Zucker, p. 69)*

71.

B. Discuss expectations related to behavior with the child. Use positive suggestions—avoid saying "Don't." Explain limits that are set on behavior before the child makes a mistake. Never threaten a child. *(Zucker, pp. 69–70)*

72.

A. Abuse is any act that is considered to be improper and that usually causes harm or pain to another. *(Zucker, p. 71)*

73.

B. All the others are frequent reasons associated with child abuse. *(Zucker, p. 72)*

74.

D. These and other reasons—for example, they don't know who to tell or they don't know any other type of behavior—are common reasons. *(Zucker, p. 72)*

75.

B. Abuse comes in many forms, especially physical, emotional, and sexual. Report any concerns you may have concerning abuse and neglect. *(Zucker, p. 72)*

76.

B. While you may be instructed to do the other things, you must report what you observe immediately! *(Zucker, p. 73)*

77.

D. Other reasons may include that the mother is unable to emotionally assume the care of the infant alone; the infant is ill. *(Zucker, p. 75)*

78.

B. Teaching by example helps to strengthen someone who can take over when you leave. *(Zucker, p. 75)*

79.

B. Most infants are fed six times a day or about every 3 to 4 hours. Nursing babies may be fed as often as every 2 hours. *(Zucker, p. 70)*

80.

B. Do not hold an infant while you are talking on the phone or cooking at the stove. *(Zucker, p. 75)*

81.

C. The mother should increase her calorie intake slightly. *(Zucker, pp. 77–78)*

82.

A. Infants should be held during bottle-feeding. Do not prop bottles. Do not leave babies unattended while they are drinking bottles. *(Zucker, p. 80)*

83.

B. Use of the dishwasher and microwave ovens is acceptable—an autoclave is not—but the most common method is on the top of the stove. *(Zucker, p. 79)*

84.

D. Begin the timing when the water comes to a full boil. *(Zucker, p. 79)*

85.

A. Concentrated liquid is the least expensive type of formula. One part concentrate is mixed with one part boiled water. *(Zucker, p. 81)*

86.

C. After two days, formula must be thrown away. *(Zucker, p. 81)*

87.

B. Disposable diapers already have protection against leakage. *(Zucker, p. 83)*

88.

A. Never pull on the cord. Let it fall off by itself. *(Zucker, p. 83)*

89.

C. This is to prevent infection. Report bleeding and discharge to your supervisor. Also keep the penis protected from rubbing on a diaper. *(Zucker, p. 84)*

90.

C. This is an indication of an infection or a sore and must be reported. *(Zucker, p. 335)*

91.

A. Casts should not cause pain. The pain should be only from the healing bone or muscle. *(Zucker, p. 335)*

92.

C. The shoulders, ankles, elbows, wrists, fingers, and toes are the most common joints affected by this disease. *(Zucker, p. 361)*

93.

A. The elderly are greatly affected by osteoarthritis, where bony surfaces become thick and develop little spurs. This causes pain every time the joint moves— the bones rub against each other, causing pain and inflammation. *(Zucker, p. 362)*

94.

B. Sometimes, a patient may appear to be getting better and concludes that he or she no longer needs the medication or may change his or her routine. This is a great mistake. *(Zucker, p. 369)*

95.

B. MS patients must be protected from exposure to infection to prevent a medical crisis. *(Zucker, p. 369)*

96.

D. Do not alter the exercise routine without discussing the change with your supervisor. *(Zucker, p. 369)*

97.

C. The immune system is compromised, and the body is no longer able to protect itself against infection. *(Zucker, p. 372)*

98.

A. This is not necessary, is very restrictive, and is most likely very uncomfortable for the patient. *(Zucker, p. 371)*

99.

B. TB patients frequently lose their appetites and will lose weight. *(Zucker, p. 370)*

100.

B. Some family members are afraid of catching TB, so they isolate or ignore the patient. Once treatment is established, the risk for family members is eliminated. *(Zucker, p. 371)*

3 Basic Needs and Body Systems

chapter objectives

Upon completion of Chapter 3, the student is responsible for the following:

➤ Define basic physical human needs.

➤ Define basic psychological human needs.

➤ Describe how to meet basic human needs.

➤ Describe family structure and function.

➤ Describe reactions to illness.

➤ Describe reactions to disabilities.

➤ Identify substance abuse.

DIRECTIONS
Each of the questions or incomplete statements below is followed by four suggested answers or completions. Select **one answer** that is best in each case.

1. Food, shelter, clothing, love, and security are best described as:
   A. psychosocial needs
   B. cultural needs
   C. spiritual needs
   D. basic needs

2. Activities of daily living (ADLs) are characterized as:
   A. physical needs
   B. cultural needs
   C. psychosocial needs
   D. spiritual needs

3. A person who needs help with his or her meals has a need for:
   A. security
   B. nourishment
   C. shelter
   D. love

4. When the home care aide provides range of motion (ROM) exercises to a patient, the aide is fulfilling the patient's need for:
   A. safety
   B. rest
   C. activity
   D. security

5. Your elderly patient enjoys visitors, especially his grandchildren. This is meeting his need for:
   A. socialization
   B. security
   C. trust
   D. shelter

6. The elderly woman you visit has a tendency to call your name loudly every time you step out of the room. When you return, she asks you to hold her hand. She may have a need for:
   A. shelter
   B. independence
   C. affection
   D. rest

7. Since becoming ill with cancer seven months ago, Miss June becomes tired very easily and requires more rest. Her food intake will be altered to balance her change in the physical need area of:
   A. clothing
   B. shelter
   C. safety
   D. activity

8. If an emotional need is not met, a person's reactions may be feelings of:
   A. anxiety
   B. depression
   C. anger
   D. all of the above

9. Reactions to pain include all of the following except:
   A. increased energy
   B. increased anxiety
   C. rapid pulse
   D. angry behavior

10. Some individual treatments of pain include hanging a charm over the bed, saying special prayers, and burning certain candles. This demonstrates differences in:
    A. countries
    B. culture
    C. physicians
    D. insurance

11. Common fear responses to pain medication include all of the following except:

    A. addiction

    B. being questioned by authorities

    C. acceptance

    D. bringing shame to families

12. An appropriate question for a home care aide to ask a patient who is in pain is:

    A. "What usually decreases your pain?"

    B. "Can I give you the pain medicine?"

    C. "Would you like for me to call the doctor?"

    D. "Why can't you think about something else?

13. Many people avoid taking pain medication, even though they are in obvious pain. How can the home care aide support a medication schedule?

    A. Offer to assist with the pain medication only when the patient complains.

    B. Encourage the patient to take the medication before the pain becomes severe.

    C. Tell the patient that you will call the doctor if the patient complains of pain.

    D. Let the patient know that you can help only when the patient becomes bedridden.

14. A unit that is bound together by common interests and working to maintain that well-being and meet the needs of all members is known as:

    A. a culture

    B. ethics

    C. a family

    D. diversity

15. Families are changing in modern times for all except which of the following reasons?

    A. Women go to work.

    B. Family members live too close to each other.

    C. People live longer.

    D. Families are smaller.

16. Descriptions of family include all of the following except:

    A. single-parent family

    B. several generations in the same house

    C. a unit of friends who live together

    D. family can only be blood relatives

17. Mr. Burke had been a farmer all his life and provided a living for his family. Now, at age 83, he is unable to care for himself and his family. His primary role was that of:

    A. son

    B. father

    C. uncle

    D. grandfather

18. The traditional description of a female caregiver includes all of the following elements except:

    A. age 45 to 50 years old

    B. mother to her children, who are often teenagers

    C. wife to her husband

    D. caring for their siblings

19. Your patient asks you, "Do you think my son should have bought that car?" Your response should be:

    A. "No, it costs too much. He should take care of you."

    B. "I'm not really in a position to comment. Discuss your feelings with your son."

    C. "He's an adult. He can do what he wants."

    D. "Yes, it's beautiful."

20. The most useful action you can take as a home care aide in response to reactions to being ill and dependent is to:

    A. involve the patient and family in the plan of care

    B. provide ADLs

    C. cook meals

    D. wash laundry

21. The absence of good health is known as:
    A. disability
    B. chronic
    C. illness
    D. acute

22. A condition that produces a physical or mental limitation is called:
    A. disability
    B. stoic
    C. illness
    D. acute

23. A disability may be produced by all of the following except:
    A. an accident
    B. an illness
    C. a birth defect
    D. a medication

24. Mr. Garren relies on his neighbor to help buy his groceries and his church members to take him to doctor appointments. This is an example of:
    A. family dynamics
    B. support systems
    C. disability
    D. culture

25. A support system in which people help one another because they want to is:
    A. an informal system
    B. a formal system
    C. a support group
    D. none of the above

26. A support system in which people help because they are paid to do so is known as:
    A. an informal system
    B. a formal system
    C. a support group
    D. none of the above

27. People who get together usually with a leader or facilitator to discuss and share similar problems make up which type of support system?
    A. informal system
    B. formal system
    C. support group
    D. none of the above

28. Mr. Tillman is a patient for whom you have cared for three years. He has just returned from a visit to the doctor, who told him that he has six months to live. Mr. Tillman says, "There really isn't anything wrong with me." This is a reaction known as:
    A. denial
    B. anger
    C. bargaining
    D. acceptance

29. Mrs. Jacobs seems very impatient today, complaining that her medicine isn't working and that you, the home care aide, aren't doing enough. Your response should include:
    A. your irritation with such an accusation
    B. a calm response
    C. your supervisor's comments about this difficult patient
    D. your resignation

30. Which of the following actions of the home care aide indicates how he or she promotes the patient's self-care?
    A. feeding the patient every meal
    B. giving the patient a washcloth to clean his or her face
    C. selecting all the patient's outfits
    D. picking out the female patient's makeup

31. The ability to function effectively and satisfactorily in society is known as:
    A. mental health
    B. mental illness
    C. caregiver role
    D. defense mechanism

32. Characteristics of mentally healthy people include all of the following except the ability to:
    A. adapt to change
    B. give and receive affection and love
    C. withdraw from responsibility
    D. tolerate stress to varying degrees

33. Mr. Allen has had schizophrenia since he was in college. This is a form of mental illness. Which of the following is true of mental illness?
    A. It is contagious.
    B. All mental illness is permanent.
    C. With treatment many people recover.
    D. People bring mental illness on themselves.

34. Mrs. Clark, a widow for 12 years, reports to you that she sees her husband every evening at bedtime. She has never mentioned this before. What should you do?
    A. Ask her what they discuss.
    B. Report this immediately to your supervisor.
    C. Call the patient's daughter.
    D. Nothing, this is normal.

35. Some signs of depression include all of the following except:
    A. increased appetite
    B. lack of activity or social interaction
    C. lack of expression in face or voice
    D. disinterest in people

36. The most important sign of substance abuse is:
    A. altered physical appearance
    B. eating more
    C. change in the person's behavior
    D. phone calls

37. Mr. Jackson lives with his 35-year old son, who is behaving in strange ways, especially today. You suspect that he has a drug habit, and you worry about Mr. Jackson. The first thing you should do is:
    A. discuss the situation with your supervisor
    B. make sure that Mr. Jackson is in no danger
    C. contact social services
    D. tell the son that he has to stop misbehaving

38. Mental changes associated with aging include:
    A. getting confused, forgetful, and dependent
    B. dementia
    C. senility
    D. none of the above

39. Social changes that the elderly experience include all of the following except:
    A. retirement
    B. change in income
    C. change in level of activity
    D. increased independence

40. The largest organ in the human body is the:
    A. heart
    B. brain
    C. lungs
    D. skin

41. The body system that acts as a framework for the body, giving it structure and support, is the:
    A. muscular system
    B. skeletal system
    C. central nervous system
    D. endocrine system

42. The parts of the body where two bones come together and there is movement are called:
    A. joints
    B. ligaments
    C. tendons
    D. bursae

43. The body system that makes all motion possible is the:
    A. circulatory system
    B. skeletal system
    C. digestive system
    D. muscular system

44. Mary is 43 years old and has had multiple sclerosis (MS) for 20 years. Her right arm is in a permanent fixed position as a result of her MS. This is called a(n):
    A. abduction
    B. adduction
    C. contracture
    D. range of motion

45. The body system that controls and organizes voluntary and involuntary body activity is the:
    A. central nervous system
    B. integumentary system
    C. circulatory system
    D. respiratory system

46. Glands that secrete hormones into the bloodstream form the:
    A. digestive system
    B. endocrine system
    C. reproductive system
    D. muscular system

47. Blood vessels leading away from the heart, such as the aorta, are known as:
    A. arteries
    B. veins
    C. capillaries
    D. atria

48. The lymphatic system, which drains fluid from body tissues, is part of the:
    A. central nervous system
    B. digestive system
    C. urinary system
    D. circulatory system

49. A very weak patient or one who is having trouble breathing must be watched very carefully while eating so that food does not get into the trachea. This is known as:
    A. digestion of food
    B. inhalation of food
    C. aspiration of food
    D. elimination of food

50. The part of the body where digestion begins is the:
    A. stomach
    B. intestines
    C. mouth
    D. liver

51. The function of the large intestine is to:
    A. begin digestion
    B. finish digestion
    C. produce bile
    D. reabsorb water into the body

52. The body system that filters out waste products and toxins from the blood is called the:
    A. digestive system
    B. urinary system
    C. respiratory system
    D. circulatory system

53. Jill is 30 years old and has had cerebral palsy since birth. This is an example of a(n):
    A. infectious disease
    B. developmental disability
    C. mental illness
    D. vitamin deficiency

54. Sherry has cerebral palsy, and she is now 6 years old. Her care plan:
    A. will be like that of other 6-year-olds
    B. will include special instruction on how to feed her
    C. will give the home care aide authority over Sherry
    D. all of the above

55. The exchange of oxygen and carbon dioxide occurs in the:
    A. bronchi
    B. trachea
    C. alveoli
    D. bronchioles

56. When your patient functions as well as possible in all areas of life, she has reached her best overall health. By encouraging her to do as much for herself as possible, you help to increase her:
    A. self-esteem
    B. blood pressure
    C. dietary intake
    D. elimination

57. Basic human needs influence behavior. To help meet the physical needs of the patients in your care, you can:
    A. finish dressing the patient when he or she is too slow
    B. keep the wheelchair brakes unlocked
    C. tell your supervisor if your patient is having difficulty breathing
    D. scold the patient if she or he spills food

58. Which organ in the female reproductive system produces the hormones estrogen and progesterone?
    A. ovaries
    B. uterus
    C. fallopian tubes
    D. vagina

59. Which body system produces hair and nails?
    A. skeletal
    B. muscular
    C. integumentary
    D. circulatory

60. Your patient's circulation tends to slow down while he is in bed. Important safety considerations include all of the following except:
    A. quickly sitting in an upright position
    B. sitting at the edge of the bed
    C. standing up and go to the bathroom
    D. all of the above

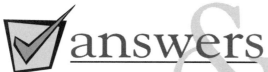

answers & rationales

1.

D. Basic needs are essential for day-to-day existence. *(Zucker, p. 33)*

2.

A. ADLs (e.g., bathing, grooming, eating) are best described as physical needs. *(Zucker, p. 33)*

3.

B. He needs help with his need for nourishment—food. *(Zucker, p. 33)*

4.

C. Activity is a basic physical need of humans. *(Zucker, p. 34)*

5.

A. Socialization helps a person to have a healthy emotional and social outlook. *(Zucker, p. 34)*

6.

C. Meeting this need helps a person's emotional health. *(Zucker, p. 34)*

7.

D. When a person is ill and requires more rest, his or her food intake must be changed to meet this change in activity—a balance of needs. *(Zucker, p. 33)*

8.

D. Or the patient may develop a physical ailment without apparent cause. *(Zucker, p. 35)*

9.

A. Actually, people in pain have increased fatigue, along with the other symptoms listed. *(Zucker, p. 35)*

10.

B. Different cultures treat pain in different ways. *(Zucker, p. 35)*

11.

C. Medication for pain is becoming more and more acceptable and available to patients at home who are in pain. *(Zucker, p. 36)*

12.

A. Do not change the patient's routine. If something works to decrease his or her pain, keep doing that. *(Zucker, p. 36)*

13.

B. By maintaining a regular schedule of pain medication, the patient may avoid episodes of severe pain that may be more difficult to treat. *(Zucker, p. 36)*

14.

C. This is an appropriate definition of family. Different cultures define family in different ways. *(Zucker, p. 37)*

15.

B. Actually, family members do not live near each other now as much as they used to. *(Zucker, p. 37)*

16.

D. Family is identified as those individuals who share common interests and goals and who regard themselves as family. *(Zucker, p. 37)*

17.

B. Traditionally, farmers and fathers provided for their families. Today, those roles are changing. *(Zucker, p. 38)*

18.

D. Most women caregivers are caring for a mother or father, who is 70 to 75 years old. *(Zucker, p. 38)*

19.

B. Act in a nonjudgmental way, and don't inflict your opinions on the patient or the patient's family. *(Zucker, p. 39)*

20.

A. Remember that you will leave but they will all remain in the home. *(Zucker, p. 40)*

21.

C. Illness is a deviation from the healthy state. *(Zucker, p. 41)*

22.

A. A disability is partial or complete loss of the use of a part or parts of the body. *(Zucker, p. 41)*

23.

D. A disability is usually permanent and is usually caused by an accident, illness, or birth defect. *(Zucker, p. 41)*

24.

B. A support system is an arrangement that gives aid and comfort to a person. *(Zucker, p. 41)*

25.

A. This is exactly what an informal support system is: church groups, neighbors, and friends. *(Zucker, p. 41)*

26.

B. These individuals may have a particular knowledge or skill level—such as a visiting nurse, home care aide, or caseworker. *(Zucker, p. 41)*

27.

C. These groups help each other and gain knowledge from each other. *(Zucker, p. 41)*

28.

A. Some people use denial when they meet a situation with which they cannot cope at the time. They say that nothing is wrong. *(Zucker, p. 42)*

29.

B. Do not take the patient's words as a personal insult. Often the patient is angry at the situation, not at you. *(Zucker, p. 41)*

30.

B. Encourage the patient to do as much for himself or herself as possible. *(Zucker, p. 43)*

31.

A. Mental health also includes a sense of well-being. It is a condition of the whole person. *(Zucker, p. 44)*

32.

C. Mentally healthy people are able to accept responsibility for their own feelings and actions. *(Zucker, p. 44)*

33.

C. In fact, they may go on to lead productive lives. Not all mental disability is permanent. *(Zucker, p. 44)*

34.

B. A classic symptom of mental illness or mental changes is a marked change in behavior patterns, which should be reported to your supervisor. *(Zucker, p. 44)*

35.

A. Actually, poor appetite is an indicator of depression as a reaction to illness. *(Zucker, p. 45)*

36.

C. This is the most significant indicator of substance abuse: a change in the person's behavior. *(Zucker, p. 47)*

37.

B. First, you must be sure that the abuser is not able to harm your patient or harm you. *(Zucker, p. 48)*

38.

D. It was once thought that all older people become senile, a condition that is now known as dementia and evidenced by confusion and forgetfulness. This is not a normal part of aging. *(Zucker, p. 56)*

39.

D. The elderly experience increased dependence upon others. Some of these changes are a result of physical changes, some are brought about by society, and some just happen. *(Zucker, p. 56)*

40.

D. It is the largest organ in the body and functions to protect us from infection, regulate temperature, and remove waste products. *(Zucker, p. 98)*

41.

B. The skeletal system is made up of more than 206 bones, giving the body shape and support. *(Zucker, p. 99)*

42.

A. Joints are areas in which one bone connects with one or more other bones. *(Zucker, p. 100)*

43.

D. The muscular system is a group of organs that allow the body to move. *(Zucker, p. 101)*

44.

C. Contracture is a permanent muscle shortening or loss of function and a permanent flexed position of the limb. *(Zucker, p. 101)*

45.

A. The brain, spinal cord, and nerves control and organize all body activity. *(Zucker, p. 102)*

46.

B. The endocrine glands secrete substances called hormones into the bloodstream, sending chemical messages to all parts of the body. *(Zucker, p. 103)*

47.

A. These vessels carry blood that is rich in oxygen to all parts of the body. *(Zucker, p. 105)*

48.

D. The lymphatic system assists the circulatory system to remove fluids away from body tissues. Lymph channels are located in the body near veins. *(Zucker, p. 106)*

49.

C. Food does not belong in the trachea or the lungs; only air does. *(Zucker, p. 107)*

50.

C. Digestion begins in the mouth, where food is chewed and mixed with saliva. *(Zucker, p. 109)*

51.

D. The large intestine, or colon, reabsorbs water into the body. Digestion is completed in the small intestine. *(Zucker, p. 109)*

52.

B. It rids the body and bloodstream of waste products and disposes of them in urine. *(Zucker, p. 109)*

53.

B. Developmental disabilities interfere with a person's proper development. *(Zucker, pp. 73–74)*

54.

B. Children with developmental disabilities have the same needs as other children but will have special instructions on the care plan on how to specially feed, carry, and ambulate the patient. *(Zucker, p. 74)*

55.

C. The alveoli, part of the respiratory system, are microscopic air sacs in the lung where oxygen passes into the blood in exchange for waste products. *(Zucker, p. 108)*

56.

A. A goal of care is to promote self-care, resulting in self-esteem and a sense of purpose. *(Zucker, p. 43)*

57.

C. Breathing—air—is a basic physical need for everyone. If the patient is having difficulty breathing, this should be reported. *(Zucker, p. 33)*

58.

A. The ovaries produce the primary female sex hormones: estrogen and progesterone. *(Zucker, p. 110)*

59.

C. Nails and hair grow from the skin. *(Zucker, p. 99)*

60.

A. Allow the patient to move carefully and slowly from a lying to a sitting position. He or she might become dizzy and faint. *(Zucker, p. 106)*

4 Mental Health and Mental Illness

chapter objectives

Upon completion of Chapter 4, the student is responsible for the following:

➤ Identify characteristics of good mental health.

➤ Identify misconceptions about mental disabilities.

➤ Describe the home care aide's role when caring for a patient who is mentally disabled.

➤ Define defense mechanisms.

➤ Identify signs of substance abuse.

DIRECTIONS Each of the questions or incomplete statements below is followed by four suggested answers or completions. Select **one answer** that is best in each case.

1. Defense mechanisms are designed to:
   A. allow the mentally ill to escape reality
   B. allow the physically ill to cope with stress
   C. assist dysfunctional individuals with reality
   D. help people to deal with stress

2. Mental disability can be caused by:
   A. chronic stress
   B. drugs
   C. isolation
   D. all of the above

3. Being able to effectively function in a certain society best defines being:
   A. socially acceptable
   B. mentally healthy
   C. culturally correct
   D. socially adaptable

4. Symptoms of mental disability include:
   A. sleeplessness
   B. decreased memory
   C. mood swings
   D. all of the above

5. Depression is best described as:
   A. mental illness
   B. a feeling of hopelessness accompanied by decreased vitality
   C. a state of relying on others for things the person is capable of doing
   D. all of the above

6. The onset of mental illness usually occurs:
   A. very rapidly and is severe
   B. very slowly with gradual behavior changes
   C. as a reaction to a traumatic life event
   D. as a result of hereditary factors

7. Mentally ill people:
   A. can be recognized by looking at their eyes
   B. can fool most of the people around them about their condition
   C. show their disability in different ways
   D. all of the above

8. Which of the following is/are true?
   A. There are many levels of mental dysfunction.
   B. Depression is a sign of mental illness.
   C. People with mental disability need to be hospitalized at least for awhile.
   D. all of the above

9. Defense mechanisms are:
   A. normally used by people when subjected to stress
   B. a sign of mental disability
   C. used by the mentally ill to protect themselves
   D. a method of accepting an unpleasant situation

10. A patient who has been diagnosed with a chronic disease may choose to not do anything and may let others take care of him. This is the defense mechanism of:
    A. repression
    B. regression
    C. projection
    D. overdependence

11. Your patient returns from her daily radiation therapy and tells you that the doctor says she doesn't need any more treatment. However, the information from your supervisor specifically asks you to have her ready at the same time the next day for more extensive radiation therapy. Your patient is using the defense mechanism of:
    A. aggression
    B. regression
    C. denial
    D. depression

12. If your patient has not told you the truth about what the doctor said about the progression of his disease, you should:
    A. tell him you know the truth and are there to listen if he needs you
    B. ask his family to make him talk to them about the situation
    C. show respect for his feelings and be supportive
    D. all of the above

13. The night after you have discovered that your favorite patient of two months is not responding well to radiation therapy and is not telling you the truth about her situation, you are unable to sleep well and do not want to return to her home. You are experiencing:
    A. denial
    B. depression
    C. hostility
    D. overdependency

14. You are very upset about your relationship with a new patient, so you put it out of your mind by spending your day off cleaning out closets and doing the yard work you had been putting off. You are using the defense mechanism of:
    A. denial
    B. depression
    C. repression
    D. hostility

15. Your patient tells you that he thinks he will discontinue his radiation therapy because he feels that it is of no use and his condition is hopeless. He is probably experiencing:
    A. depression
    B. regression
    C. projection
    D. rationalization

16. Your patient's four-year-old son has started bedwetting and sucking his thumb again since his mother came home with his new baby brother. He is going through:
    A. depression
    B. regression
    C. aggression
    D. repression

17. Depression can be:
    A. an illness
    B. a way in which a person deals with an illness
    C. a side effect of medication
    D. all of the above

18. Your 57-year-old male patient has been diagnosed with lung cancer. He is very angry and says that if his wife had quit smoking, he would have, too, and he would not be sick. He is using the defense mechanism of:
    A. denial
    B. projection
    C. aggression
    D. repression

19. Your patient asks you to get some bug spray for the bugs that are all over the walls in her bedroom. She is pointing to the walls, but you do not see any bugs, so you should:
    A. contact your supervisor immediately
    B. not allow your patient to take her scheduled medication until you have talked with your supervisor
    C. ask the patient how long she has been seeing bugs on the wall
    D. all of the above

20. If your patient is mentally ill, the care you give will:
    A. be very similar to what you give to physically ill patients
    B. require that you know how to apply restraints
    C. be prescribed by a psychologist
    D. all of the above

21. The patient's plan of care states that you are to provide an accepting environment. This means that you will need to:
    A. accept the patient's decisions about his or her care
    B. arrange the bedroom furniture to the patient's preference
    C. be accepting of the patient but not necessarily of his or her actions
    D. all of the above

22. You can best help others to feel positive about the patient who is mentally ill by:
    A. using a friendly, understanding manner when caring for the patient
    B. using childlike terms when talking to the patient
    C. taking care of the patient's personal hygiene needs yourself
    D. all of the above

23. Mentally ill patients may have difficulty:
    A. adapting to change
    B. giving and receiving affection and love
    C. distinguishing between reality and unreality
    D. all of the above

24. When caring for a depressed person, it is important that you:
    A. understand that some patients will remain depressed no matter what you do
    B. realize that the patient's safety becomes more of a responsibility
    C. report any changes in the patient's behavior or mood to your supervisor
    D. all of the above

25. A family member tells you that your patient with a mental illness is in the bedroom acting crazy and that you must do something now. You should:
    A. lock the bedroom door
    B. notify your supervisor immediately
    C. check the chart to see whether the family member can give the patient a medication
    D. All of the above

26. A family member of your patient with a mental illness says that you need to make him stop acting crazy. Your best response is to:
    A. laugh as though the family member were making a joke and continue with your work
    B. use body language to show your disapproval of the comment and continue your work
    C. ask the family member whether she has any suggestions as to how you would do that
    D. ask the family member what the patient is doing and report her comments to your supervisor

27. Your patient appears confused and is packing a suitcase to leave. You should:
    A. hold the patient by the hand so that he cannot leave
    B. with the family's help, use a sheet to restraint the patient in a chair
    C. lock the bedroom door
    D. none of the above

28. Mental disability may be caused by:
    A. drug and alcohol abuse
    B. personality changes
    C. being overly indulged as a child
    D. none of the above

29. Family members seem uncomfortable with your patient's behavior and are not coming to visit as often as they did. As a result, your patient seems more depressed and withdrawn. You should:
    A. tell the family about the situation so that they can visit more
    B. encourage the family to get professional help so that they can deal with the patient
    C. share your observations with your supervisor
    D. all of the above

30. If your patient is abusing drugs, which of the following is/are true?
    A. It is best that the family not confront her.
    B. If the family members continue to show love for her, she will get control of the habit.

C. Her behavior will begin to show definite changes.

D. all of the above

31. Signs of substance abuse include:

A. using a sleeping pill to get to sleep

B. disinterest in familiar activities

C. more agreeable personality

D. all of the above

32. General misconceptions about substance abuse include:

A. Everyone does it.

B. I can control the habit.

C. No one will know I'm doing it.

D. all of the above

33. If you suspect that your patient is abusing drugs or alcohol, what would be the most significant sign?

A. The patient's behavior changes.

B. The patient's interest in familiar activities changes.

C. Relationships within the family change.

D. The patient's level of energy changes.

34. If you are assigned to care for a patient who has a drug abuser or alcoholic in the home, your major responsibility is to:

A. have the family seek the appropriate help

B. make sure the patient is safe

C. prepare detailed reports of all of the abuser's comments

D. all of the above

35. If you think your patient is abusing alcohol, you should:

A. discuss the problems that alcohol can cause

B. tell the family in a nice way that you cannot be responsible for the patient's safety

C. share any change in gait, breath odor, or physical appearance with your supervisor

D. all of the above

36. If your patient has a history of alcoholism and the family has done nothing to change it, you should:

A. make the family feel guilty about letting the drinking continue

B. call and ask members of Alcoholics Anonymous to come to the house

C. use nonjudgmental behavior and let your supervisor develop a plan

D. all of the above

37. The patient is considered a drug abuser when:

A. the drug causes adverse consequences that affect major life areas

B. the drug alters the patient's mental or physical state

C. the patient uses the drug to avoid pain

D. the drug is used to alter the patient's body's responses

38. Some of the known causes of mental retardation include all of the following except:

A. genetic defects

B. traumatic brain injury

C. proper prenatal care

D. drug addiction of the mother

39. A basic principle in treatment of the mentally retarded involves incorporating the individual into regular activities. This is called:

A. mainstreaming

B. sundowning

C. normalization

D. rationalization

40. Major goals of a treatment plan for mentally retarded individuals include all of the following except:

A. promoting the physical health of the individual

B. developing motor functions and activities of daily living

C. encouraging and developing communication skills

D. isolating them from the external social world

41. Characteristics of mental health include:
    A. giving and accepting love and affection
    B. anger, frustration, and anxiety
    C. extended depression after losses
    D. blaming others for one's disappointments

42. Abilities that demonstrate an individual's mental health include all of the following except:
    A. adapting and adjusting to change
    B. accepting and handling responsibility for one's decisions, feelings, and actions
    C. dealing with reality in a helpful way
    D. spending one's paycheck on the lottery out of frustration

43. Patients with mental illnesses are encouraged and counseled to be able to make their own decisions. This is known as:
    A. self-reliance
    B. autonomy
    C. depression
    D. normalization

44. Behavior that is inappropriate to the life situation is known as:
    A. mental health
    B. mental illness
    C. mental retardation
    D. mental hygiene

45. Common symptoms of mental illness include all of the following except:
    A. increased appetite
    B. fatigue
    C. insomnia
    D. apathy

46. When a patient has feelings of extreme sadness—feeling dejected and discouraged—he or she is experiencing:
    A. aggression
    B. denial
    C. depression
    D. projection

47. Refusing to believe the truth about something is known as:
    A. aggression
    B. denial
    C. depression
    D. projection

48. Putting an unpleasant or painful feeling out of your mind is called:
    A. projection
    B. rationalization
    C. regression
    D. repression

49. Myths about mental illness include all except which of the following?
    A. Mentally ill people have lost their minds.
    B. Mentally ill people cannot work.
    C. Mentally ill people are dangerous.
    D. Mentally ill people can get better.

50. As you provide care and support to Mrs. Kline while she is being treated for clinical depression, you should report which of the following observations to your supervisor?
    A. Mrs. Kline is able to feed herself.
    B. Mrs. Kline refuses to take her antidepressant medication.
    C. Mrs. Kline assists with her bathing.
    D. Mrs. Kline speaks to her sister on the phone twice a day.

51. Your patient tells you that he would like to die and has the gun to do it. Your response to this would include:
    A. telling him not to talk like that
    B. allowing him to talk about his feelings
    C. demanding that he give you the gun
    D. telling him that you don't blame him for wanting to end a life of pain and misery

52. Mr. Maloney has been ill with clinical depression for many years and has shown signs of improvement, only to become ill again. Recently, he has been insisting that you perform all of his ADLs as well as feed him, answer his phone calls, and read to him, although he is able to do these things for himself. This patient is showing signs of:
   A. denial
   B. overdependence
   C. aggression
   D. projection

53. The primary sign of depression is:
   A. increased appetite
   B. lack of any interest in the present situation
   C. participation in social activities
   D. laughter and smiling

54. The role of the home care aide in providing care for the patient with depression includes all of the following except:
   A. encouraging the patient's decisions and opinions
   B. allowing the patient to take part in as much self-care as he or she is able to
   C. establishing successful routines
   D. avoiding talking to the patient

55. While shopping at the grocery store for your family, you see the caregiver of your patient, who says that she just had to get out of the house, leaving the patient alone. What should you do with this information?
   A. Immediately go to the patient's house.
   B. Call the police.
   C. Report this information to your supervisor.
   D. Take the caregiver to the hospital.

56. You provide care for a woman who has manic depression and severe mood swings. She tells you, "It's not my fault that I have this problem. It's the doctor's fault." This is an example of what kind of defense mechanism?
   A. projection
   B. regression
   C. repression
   D. aggression

57. The defense mechanism of acting like a child or becoming very dependent is known as:
   A. projection
   B. regression
   C. repression
   D. aggression

58. Hallucinations, disorientation, and forgetfulness are symptoms of:
   A. mental health
   B. mental disability
   C. mental hygiene
   D. none of the above

59. Which of the following myths is associated with mental illness and disability?
   A. Mental disabilities are contagious.
   B. Not all disability is permanent.
   C. Patients with mental disability should not be labeled.
   D. There are many causes for mental disabilities.

60. As a home care aide, you demonstrate mental health by:
   A. reporting to work on time for each assignment
   B. showing anger when your patient curses at you
   C. yelling back at a verbally abusive patient
   D. all of the above

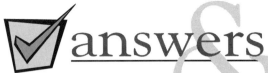
1.

D. A defense mechanism is a thought that is used unconsciously to protect oneself against painful or unpleasant feelings. *(Zucker, p. 45)*

2.

D. Mental disability is a permanent or temporary disruption in a person's ability to function satisfactorily in society. All of these things can cause a temporary or permanent disruption in the ability to function. *(Zucker, p. 44)*

3.

B. Mental health refers to the ability to function satisfactorily in a society. None of the other choices describes mental health. *(Zucker, p. 44)*

4.

D. When a person cannot function satisfactorily in society, he or she may exhibit sleeplessness, decreased memory, and mood swings. *(Zucker, p. 45)*

5.

B. Depression may be a defense mechanism, an illness, the result or an illness, or the side effect of medications. Its primary sign is a lack of any interest in the situation and environment. *(Zucker, p. 45)*

6.

B. Mental disability may be caused by heredity or as a reaction to a traumatic event, but it usually develops slowly with gradual changes in ability to function. *(Zucker, p. 44)*

7.

C. Different people who show their disability in different ways, showing marked changes in behavior patterns. People's eyes may mirror their stress or anxiety but are not diagnostic of mental illness. Mentally ill people are not trying to fool others. *(Zucker, p. 44)*

8.

A. Mental dysfunction can range from the overuse of defense mechanisms to loss of contact with reality. Depression is not necessarily related to mental illness but can be triggered by medications and other things. Hospitalization is not required for all people with mental disabilities. *(Zucker, p. 44)*

9.

A. All people use defense mechanisms to protect themselves against painful or unpleasant feelings. They are not used just by the mentally ill, nor are they a sign of acceptance or disability. *(Zucker, p. 45)*

10.

D. When some people realize that they are no longer in total charge of their situation, they are unable to adjust to the change and react by giving others complete responsibility for their care. Repression, regression, and projection are all types of defense mechanisms. *(Zucker, pp. 45–46)*

11.

C. People who are in denial simply refuse to believe what is happening. Other choices are different defense mechanisms. *(Zucker, p. 45)*

12.

C. It is not your role to confront the patient or force the patient to talk about the situation. Your role is to treat the patient with respect, support the patient and his or her family, see to the patient's safety, and follow the plan of care. *(Zucker, p. 44)*

13.

B. Depression can be a defense mechanism, which you are using to protect yourself against painful or unpleasant feelings. *(Zucker, p. 45)*

14.

C. When you put it out of your mind, you are using repression as a defense mechanism to protect yourself against painful or unpleasant feelings. You are not using denial, because you acknowledge that the situation exists. You are active, not depressed, and you are not angry or hostile. *(Zucker, p. 45)*

15.

A. Feelings of hopelessness are typical of depression. Use of regression means that she would act like a child; use of projection means that she would blame others for the problem; use of rationalization means that she would make excuses for unacceptable behavior. *(Zucker, p. 45)*

16.

B. Because he is threatened by his new brother, he is reverting to behavior that he used when he was younger. *(Zucker, p. 45)*

17.

D. All of these situations can result in depression. Depression can be an illness of itself. A person who is diagnosed with a serious illness may use depression as a defense mechanism for a time. Some medications can cause depression as a side effect. *(Zucker, p. 45)*

18.

B. Projection is a defense mechanism in which someone else is blamed for a situation. Other choices are different types of defense mechanisms. *(Zucker, p. 45)*

19.

A. When a patient is seeing things that are not there, it is important to report this change in behavior and senses immediately. It is not within your role to withhold a medication nor to attempt to get more information about the hallucination from the patient. *(Zucker, p. 46)*

20.

A. A patient is mentally ill still has the same needs as a person who is mentally healthy. Your role is to meet those physical and safety needs, just as you would for any other patient. You will not be applying restraints or receiving orders from a psychologist. *(Zucker, p. 46)*

21.

C. The patient may not necessarily be able to make decisions about his or her care. You are to be accepting of the patient, even though you may not be accepting of inappropriate behavior. *(Zucker, p. 46)*

22.

A. When you exhibit genuine caring, friendliness, and understanding of a mentally ill patient, you are modeling accepting behavior for others. *(Zucker, p. 46)*

23.

D. All of us may, at times, have difficulty with these areas. Mentally ill patients are able to do all of these things but will have more difficulty with them than others would. *(Zucker, p. 44)*

24.

D. All of these actions are appropriate to take when caring for a depressed patient. You may not be able to see any positive changes in the patient's level of depression. You may need to be more aware of safety issues because the patient may no longer care about danger to himself or herself. You should report any changes in the depressed patient's mood or behavior because such changes may be significant. *(Zucker, p. 45)*

25.

B. Any time a patient's behavior changes, you should immediately notify your supervisor, who will evaluate the situation. It is not your role to restrain the patient in a locked room or tell the family to give the patient medications. *(Zucker, p. 46)*

26.

D. You need to report objectively what the patient is doing, not simply that he or she is "acting crazy." Obtain this information from the family member and relay it to your supervisor. It is not appropriate for you to ignore the family's crisis or ask for their advice on how to handle the situation. *(Zucker, p. 46)*

27.

D. A mentally ill patient still has rights. You cannot restrain the client in any way without an order to do so. *(Zucker, p. 5)*

28.

A. Alcohol and drugs can interfere with the brain's ability to process input and information, causing mental disability. This may be a temporary or permanent condition. Personality changes and childhood indulgence are not considered causes of mental disability. *(Zucker, p. 44)*

29.

C. Your observations about the patient and his or her family are very important. The family must have support to be supportive of the patient. It is not in your role to tell family members to change their behavior, but it is appropriate for you to share your observations with your supervisor. *(Zucker, p. 46)*

30.

C. Many signs are associated with substance abuse. The most important sign is a change in the person's behavior. A plan must be made to deal with the situation, including confrontation and showing support. *(Zucker, p. 47)*

31.

B. This is a sign of substance abuse because the abuser becomes interested only in the drug and its effects.

Using a sleeping pill may or may not indicate abuse, and a more agreeable personality is not usually indicative of substance abuse. *(Zucker, p. 47)*

32.

D. All of these are misconceptions about substance abuse because they allow the abuser to rationalize or pretend to be in control of the situation. *(Zucker, p. 47)*

33.

A. This is the most important sign of substance abuse; the other signs may not develop until later in the dependency process. Observing changes in behavior early and reporting them helps promote early intervention. *(Zucker, p. 47)*

34.

B. Your primary responsibility is to the patient. A plan must be made to offer help to the abuser, so make your supervisor aware of the situation. A detailed report of the abuser's comments would not be helpful in dealing with this situation. *(Zucker, p. 48)*

35.

C. In this way you are reporting objective information to your supervisor. Other choices do not give objective information and are not appropriate for this problem. *(Zucker, p. 49)*

36.

C. The family members may not know what to do, but with the help and support of you and your supervisor, a plan can be made. *(Zucker, p. 49)*

37.

A. Substance abuse is the use of anything, usually drugs or alcohol, to an excess and to the detriment of the person and his or her life. Most drugs alter physical and mental states but are not abused unless they affect the patient adversely in major life areas. *(Zucker, p. 46)*

38.

C. Poor prenatal care is a known cause of mental retardation, along with the others listed. *(Model Curriculum, p. 162)*

39.

C. Normalization as a basic principle means that the mentally retarded individual should have as normal an existence as possible. *(Model Curriculum, p. 162)*

40.

D. A goal includes developing their ability to function in the social environment. *(Model Curriculum, p. 163)*

41.

A. Giving and accepting love and affection is a significant characteristic of mental health. *(Model Curriculum, p. 180)*

42.

D. A characteristic of mental health is the ability to control desires and impulses until they can be fulfilled appropriately. *(Model Curriculum, p. 180)*

43.

B. Autonomy is making one's own decisions; this is of particular importance to those with disabilities and illnesses. *(Model Curriculum, p. 181)*

44.

B. This is the definition of mental illness. The individual is not able to function at a high level in the family, the home, or the community. *(Model Curriculum, p. 181)*

45.

A. Anorexia, or lack of appetite, is a common symptom of mental illness when clustered with the others listed. *(Model Curriculum, p. 182)*

46.

C. Depression is extreme sadness; the person feels dejected and discouraged, and it is shown by feelings of hopelessness, helplessness, and despair. *(Model Curriculum, p. 183)*

47.

B. Denial is a way of adapting in which a person refuses to believe that something is or can be disturbing. *(Model Curriculum, p. 183)*

48.

D. Repression is a tool that is commonly used to put out of the mind feelings and events that are unpleasant and painful. *(Model Curriculum, p. 184)*

49.

D. One of the myths is that mentally ill people will never get better. In fact, many are cured of their illness and are quite functional. *(Model Curriculum, p. 185)*

50.

B. You should report any change in patient behaviors, especially those that are detrimental to the patient's health. *(Model Curriculum, p. 186)*

51.

B. If you feel comfortable doing it, allow the patient to talk about such feelings while you listen patiently and caringly. *(Model Curriculum, p. 187)*

52.

B. When a patient does not assume the responsibility that he or she is able to take, the patient is said to be overdependent. *(Zucker, p. 46)*

53.

B. Depression is low spirits that may or may not cause a change of activity. The primary sign of depression is lack of any interest in the present situation and the present environment. *(Zucker, p. 45)*

54.

D. Communicate and encourage the patient with depression. Be patient and supportive. Remember that some patients will remain depressed no matter what you do. *(Zucker, p. 46)*

55.

C. Should you find out information about the patient's care, report your observations objectively to your supervisor. *(Zucker, p. 43)*

56.

A. Projection is placing the blame on others or putting one's own feelings on others. *(Zucker, p. 45; Model Curriculum, p. 183)*

57.

B. Regression is going back in one's mind to think and act like a much younger person or like a child. *(Zucker, p. 45: Model Curriculum, p. 183)*

58.

B. Mental disability includes these symptoms and others; it is the permanent or temporary disruption in the ability of a person to function satisfactorily in society. *(Zucker, p. 45)*

59.

A. Mental illnesses and disabilities cannot be spread through direct or indirect contact. *(Zucker, p. 44)*

60.

A. Being able to accept responsibility for your own feelings and actions is a sign of mental health. *(Zucker, p. 44)*

5 Death and Dying

chapter objectives

Upon completion of Chapter 5, the student is responsible for the following:

➤ Identify steps in the dying process.

➤ Describe the emotional needs of the dying.

➤ Describe physical care of the dying patient and family.

➤ Define postmortem care.

DIRECTIONS
Each of the questions or incomplete statements below is followed by four suggested answers or completions. Select **one answer** that is best in each case.

1. The person responsible for telling a person that he or she is dying is the:
   A. registered nurse
   B. physician
   C. clergy
   D. closest relative

2. If a family decides that a patient should not know that he or she is dying, you should:
   A. respect the family's wishes
   B. tell your supervisor to replace you as it is too difficult to keep up a lie
   C. discuss it with the family and help them see it is not fair to the patient or you
   D. tell your patient and have him keep it a secret between the two of you

3. Your supervisor informs you that the family has told the patient that he only has about three months left to live. When you arrive in the home and ask the patient how his day is going, he says, "Very good, thank you." The patient may be experiencing which stage identified by Dr. Elisabeth Kubler-Ross?
   A. depression
   B. anger
   C. bargaining
   D. denial

4. Which of the following statements is not true about the stages of dying as presented by Dr. Kubler-Ross?
   A. Everyone does not experience every step.
   B. The steps are progressive so patients go from the first step to the last.
   C. Patients are different as they try to deal with death.
   D. Members of the dying person's family also experience the stages.

5. Which of the following statements best describes a patient in the stage of denial?
   A. "I have not been feeling that bad."
   B. "I just don't want to get up today."
   C. "If I eat right and go to church, maybe I will get better."
   D. "The bad stuff always happens to me."

6. Which of the following statements best indicates a patient in the stage of anger?
   A. "I have not been feeling that bad."
   B. "I just don't want to get up today."
   C. "If I eat right and go to church, maybe I will get better."
   D. "The bad stuff always happens to me."

7. If you are uncomfortable when a patient asks you a question about dying, you should:
   A. complete the patient's care quickly so that you won't have to stay and be uncomfortable
   B. be talkative so that the patient will not guess that you are uncomfortable
   C. be honest and find the answer to the question
   D. say that it is too personal so the patient should talk to his or her family about it

8. Which of the following is *not* an emotional need of the dying patient?
   A. to have recreation
   B. to be safe and secure
   C. to experience meaningful relationships
   D. to receive assurance that he or she can get better

9. An appropriate attitude for the home care aide who is caring for a terminally ill patient is:
   A. that dying people must make peace with God

B. that each person is an individual with unique needs

C. a sense of detachment from the dying patient is needed for self-protection

D. all of the above

10. When a terminally ill patient is making seemingly unreasonable requests and complaining about everything, he or she needs:

A. to have to write out his requests on paper so that he or she can see that they are not reasonable

B. to know that people will become too uncomfortable and not want to be with him or her

C. a good listener

D. all of the above

11. One of the best ways to relate to a dying patient is to:

A. allow him to do as much as possible for himself

B. tell the patient not to worry

C. help the patient to plan his or her funeral

D. not let the patient refuse treatment and give up

12. Hospice was designed to:

A. provide the dying patient with hospital care

B. provide care for terminally ill patients in their homes

C. provide home care and family support for a terminally ill person

D. provide home care for those who cannot afford hospitalization

13. A hospice program:

A. provides support for the family after the death of their loved one

B. considers the patient and the family as a unit of care

C. makes use of a team of professionals

D. all of the above

14. Which of the following statements is true about establishing a routine for the care of a terminally ill patient?

A. Having the same schedule each day may be comforting.

B. A set schedule may not be possible because of pain and sleeping patterns of the dying.

C. Allow the patient to determine the schedule of activities for as long as possible.

D. all of the above

15. When death is near and the patient seems unconscious, you should remember to:

A. tell the patient before touching or moving him or her

B. ask whether the family wants the priest or clergy called

C. stay out of the patient's bedroom so that the family can have privacy

D. all of the above

16. Your patient tells you that the doctor is stopping the chemotherapy and she will probably only live a month or so. Your first reply would be:

A. "Don't you give up just because of that one doctor."

B. "That is upsetting. What are your feelings right now?"

C. "Can I call someone to stay with you?"

D. "There are new cures found every day so don't get depressed"

17. The day your patient tells you that the doctor is stopping his treatments and he will only live a month or so, you go home and go straight to bed without even eating supper. You are experiencing:

A. anger

B. denial

C. depression

D. association

18. When turning a terminally ill patient from his back to one side, you notice blotchy dark blue areas on the back, buttocks, and legs. You should:

    A. suspect abuse and call the police

    B. notify your supervisor and turn the patient more frequently

    C. notify your supervisor and tell the patient's family that the end is near

    D. turn the patient from side to side and not on his back

19. Your terminally ill patient says that she knows the end is near and doesn't want anything to eat or for people to bother her anymore. You should:

    A. allow the patient to do as much for herself as possible

    B. work to find ways to maintain nutrition for as long as possible

    C. have the family decide what should be done

    D. talk with your supervisor about any changes that should be made in the care plan

20. A terminally ill patient is losing strength and says that he is full after eating only a few bites of food. You should:

    A. provide small, frequent feedings

    B. tell him that he must eat to keep up his strength

    C. use carbonated and caffeinated drinks to stimulate his appetite

    D. all of the above

21. Your patient has a DNR tag on his chart. This means that:

    A. the patient does not wish to be fed by artificial means

    B. the patient has requested no resuscitation

    C. the doctor has ordered that no medical procedures be used if the patient's heart stops or he stops breathing

    D. caregivers should not reveal the fact that the patient is terminal

22. Irregular noisy breathing that stops for periods of up to 30 seconds or more is:

    A. Cheyne-Stokes respirations

    B. obstructive pulmonary disease

    C. autonomic respiratory distress

    D. dyspnea

23. Caring for the body after death includes:

    A. inserting dentures

    B. bathing the body

    C. closing the eyes but not pressing on the eyeballs

    D. all of the above

24. Care provided to the body after death is called:

    A. premortuary care

    B. TLC

    C. postmortem care

    D. terminal care

25. If the family wants to stay at the bedside with the body, you should:

    A. prepare the body appropriately then allow them to come in

    B. allow the family to stay and not be concerned about doing anything to the body

    C. explain that the family will be allowed to view the body at the funeral home

    D. tell the family that you must do a lot of things before rigor mortis sets in

26. A general policy for the removal of tubes from the patient's body is:

    A. do not remove any tubes from the body

    B. do not remove any tube from the body that you did not care for before

    C. remove all tubes and dispose of properly

    D. follow the protocol established by your agency

27. Positioning of the patient's body after death involves:

    A. removing all but one pillow from under the head

B. placing the body flat on its back

C. folding the arms across the abdomen

D. all of the above

28. All jewelry on the deceased patient should be:

A. removed and given to the spouse or oldest relative

B. identified on the chart and have the family decide what should be left on the body

C. taped in place so that it will not fall off

D. removed, tagged, and put in a safe place of the family's choosing

29. When your patient dies, a family member becomes so overcome with grief that she is screaming uncontrollably. You should first:

A. allow the other family members to care for her

B. give her one of the deceased's nerve pills

C. ask a family member to slap her gently on the cheeks

D. ask her what you can do for her so that she will not keep bothering others

30. When caring for a patient with a terminal illness who expresses concern about dying, the home care aide should:

A. tell the patient, "everything's going to be all right"

B. listen to the patient and encourage the patient to share his or her feelings

C. change the subject

D. call your supervisor

31. Hospice care is:

A. focused only on the dying patient

B. a program of care for dying hospital patients

C. a cure for terminal illness

D. a special program of care for dying patients and their families

32. To comfort a patient who is dying, the home care aide should:

A. isolate the person from the family

B. avoid discussing death

C. be there and listen

D. discuss her feelings about death

33. Denial, anger, bargaining, depression, and acceptance are identified as:

A. standard precautions

B. signs of mental illness

C. evidence of menopause

D. stages of emotions of death and dying

34. A terminally ill patient says that she plans to live long enough to see the birth of her first grandchild, due in six months. This illustrates:

A. denial

B. anger

C. bargaining

D. acceptance

35. Attitudes about death:

A. do not vary as a person ages

B. need not be identified by the home care aide

C. are the same in every culture

D. are influenced by religion

36. Before providing care to dying patients, it is important that the home care aide:

A. has experienced the death of a loved one

B. learn about medications that help to ease pain

C. understand his or her own feelings about death

D. has worked in a nursing home

37. One of the last functions to be lost is the sense of:

A. hearing

B. sight

C. taste

D. smell

38. Mouth care of terminally ill patients will include:
    A. cleansing mucous membranes with glycerine swabs as needed
    B. mouthwash three times a day
    C. brushing teeth with baking soda and peroxide
    D. all of the above

39. Children are able to understand death at which period?
    A. infancy
    B. toddler period
    C. preschool period
    D. preadolescent period

40. Mr. Nance has terminal cancer, but his family does not want to tell him. The home care aide should:
    A. tell Mr. Nance how serious his illness is
    B. tell Mr. Nance that he is going to get better
    C. respect the wishes of the family
    D. refuse to care for this patient

41. When a patient is dying, the family should be:
    A. encouraged to speak and touch him or her as usual
    B. discouraged from providing any personal care
    C. asked to leave when more than three are present
    D. encouraged to whisper and tiptoe in the patient's room

42. Which of the following is not a sign that death has occurred?
    A. no pulse
    B. the death rattle
    C. no respirations
    D. no blood pressure

43. Mouth care for the dying patient is:
    A. done only if the patient appears uncomfortable
    B. not necessary because the patient is not eating

C. done frequently because secretions tend to build up
    D. not done because it is painful

44. Patients who are in the stage of denial:
    A. are sad and quiet
    B. are angry
    C. refuse to believe they are dying
    D. make "deals" with God

45. A dying patient is talking to you about dying. What is the appropriate response?
    A. Reassure the patient that he or she is not dying.
    B. Listen and allow the patient to express his or her feelings.
    C. Tell the patient that you can't discuss this.
    D. Tell the patient that he or she will get better.

46. If the dying patient's throat contains excessive mucus secretions, the home care aide should:
    A. suction the patient
    B. ask the family to suction the patient
    C. ask for medication to be given to the patient
    D. elevate the head of the bed or prop the patient up on pillows

47. The stage of dying at which the terminally ill patient may express unwillingness to accept his or her condition is called:
    A. denial
    B. bargaining
    C. depression
    D. acceptance

48. All of the following are characteristic of the dying patient's respirations except:
    A. slow
    B. irregular
    C. fast
    D. difficult

49. Postmortem care is best described as:
    A. care before death
    B. care after death

C. comfort measures

D. care during the dying process

50. In which of the following positions is the body of the deceased placed?

A. supine

B. prone

C. Fowler's

D. semi-Fowler's

51. All of the following tasks are included in postmortem care except:

A. personal care

B. leaving the eyes open

C. folding the arms over the abdomen

D. place one pillow under the head

52. What should be done with the dentures of a deceased person?

A. remove them and place into a denture cup

B. place them in the mouth if possible

C. place them in a cup with mouthwash

D. give them to the family

53. Needs of the dying patient include all of the following except:

A. the need to be normal

B. the need to experience pain for past wrongs

C. the need for love

D. the need for recreation

54. Essential concepts in hospice care include all of the following except

A. dealing with the patient and family separately

B. using trained professionals to comfort and care for the dying

C. helping the family after the death of their loved one

D. allowing the patient as much choice as possible

55. Evidence that the circulation of a dying patient is slowing includes:

A. red extremities

B. warm toes

C. cold hands and arms

D. all of the above

56. As the moment of death nears, the patient's family requests that everyone present pray. The home care aide should:

A. respect their wishes and provide for privacy

B. begin to pray out loud

C. tell them that this is not part of her job

D. call her own spiritual leader

57. After your patient dies, his family invites you to attend the funeral. You should:

A. decline because they are of a different religion than you

B. attend as your supervisor or schedule permits

C. offer to cook a meal for all participants

D. none of the above

58. In considering the steps in the dying process, all except which of the following are true?

A. All patients are different.

B. Everyone will experience every step.

C. The family of the dying patient will go through the steps.

D. Patients do not go through these steps in any given order.

59. The dying patient wants to speak with friends and family members about his or her life. The is an example of:

A. the need to be normal

B. the need for meaningful relations

C. the need for recreation

D. the need for safety and security

60. Mrs. Oran has terminal lung cancer. She likes to spend her time awake playing cards, watching her favorite soap operas, and reading books. This is an example of:

A. the need to be normal

B. the need for meaningful relations

C. the need for recreation

D. the need for safety and security

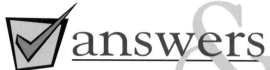

answers & rationales

1.

B. The physician is the one who determines that the patient is dying and then must decide, usually in consultation with the family, whether the patient should be told or not. The other individuals may be asked by the physician to tell the patient. *(Zucker, p. 89)*

2.

A. You are obligated to follow the family's wishes, even when you find this difficult to do. *(Zucker, p. 89)*

3.

D. Denial is the stage of not dealing with a stressful situation. *(Zucker, p. 90)*

4.

B. The steps are not progressive for every individual. *(Zucker, p. 89)*

5.

A. Denial is the stage of not believing the stressful situation. *(Zucker, p. 90)*

6.

D. Anger is the "why me?" stage. *(Zucker, p. 90)*

7.

C. Being honest and finding an answer is your responsibility. *(Zucker, p. 90)*

8.

D. The dying patient should not be offered false hope or reassurance, but be careful not to destroy hope. *(Zucker, p. 91)*

9.

B. Each person is a unique individual, even when dying. *(Zucker, p. 87)*

10.

C. A good listener can better manage unreasonable requests and complaints. *(Zucker, p. 90)*

11.

A. This permits him to be independent for as long as he is able. *(Zucker, p. 92)*

12.

C. Hospice provides care for the patient and support for the family. *(Zucker, p. 91)*

13.

D. A hospice program does all of the identified activities. *(Zucker, p. 91)*

14.

D. All of these special emotional needs are important in caring for a terminally ill patient. *(Zucker, p. 91)*

15.

A. Hearing is usually the last sense to be lost when a person is dying. *(Zucker, p. 93)*

16.

B. Asking what the patient is feeling as an initial response shows that you care. *(Zucker, p. 91)*

17.

C. Depression can be a normal reaction to a stressful situation until you are ready to deal with the situation. *(Model Curriculum, p. 195)*

18.

B. The bluish discoloring is due to stasis of the blood in the person who is very close to dying. *(Zucker, p. 93)*

19.

D. This is the patient's decision, and you must accept it, even if it is hard. Talk with your supervisor about the situation. It is inappropriate for you to force nutrition or action on your patient and her family. *(Zucker, p. 91)*

20.

A. Offer frequent sips of water and small feedings so as not to tire the patient with long meals. It is not appropriate to urge additional food or drinks on the patient. *(Zucker, p. 93)*

21.

C. DNR stands for "do not resuscitate." This must be ordered by a doctor after discussion with the patient while the patient is able to understand the decision and its consequences. *(Zucker, p. 92)*

22.

A. This type of respiration may be upsetting to observe but is a very usual occurrence as patients approach death. It is a specific pattern of breathing, not a respiratory disease or difficulty in breathing. *(Zucker, p. 93)*

23.

D. All of these actions are taken in caring for the body after death to prepare it for removal. These actions help the patient to look clean and at peace if the family wishes to see the body. *(Zucker, p. 94)*

24.

C. "Post" means after, and "mortem" means death in Latin. *(Zucker, p. 94)*

25.

A. After death occurs, the family may want to sit at the bedside and say their final goodbyes. Prepare the body for removal first, then allow the family to come in. In this way, the patient will look more natural and at peace when the family members view the body. *(Zucker, p. 94)*

26.

D. Each agency has established policies regarding removal of tubes after death. These may vary with the circumstances of the death, so always follow policy. *(Zucker, p. 94)*

27.

D. All of these choices are appropriate in positioning a patient after death. This prepares the body for removal to the funeral home. *(Zucker, p. 94)*

28.

B. Identified on the chart and have the family decide what should be left on the body. *(Zucker, p. 94)*

29.

A. Ask the family how you can help, and try to do whatever is necessary to help them through this difficult time. *(Zucker, p. 94)*

30.

B. Don't offer false hope or reassurance. Be a good listener, and encourage expression of feelings. *(Zucker, p. 91)*

31.

D. Hospice care is a program of care that allows a dying patient to remain at home and die at home while receiving professionally supervised care. *(Zucker, p. 91)*

32.

C. Be a good listener. It is one of the best things a home care aide can do for any patient. *(Zucker, p. 90)*

33.

D. These are the stages or steps experienced by people who are dying. *(Zucker, p. 90)*

34.

C. Bargaining is characterized by making promises to do something special or to change his or her life if the dying person is allowed to continue living. *(Model Curriculum, p. 195)*

35.

D. Adult attitudes toward death and dying are influenced by background, culture, and religion. *(Model Curriculum, p. 195)*

36.

C. There is no right or wrong way to feel about death, but you should be aware of your own feelings and thoughts. *(Zucker, p. 92)*

37.

A. Hearing is the last sense to be lost. Talk openly and compassionately to a dying patient. *(Zucker, p. 93)*

38.

A. Mouth care may include cleansing with glycerine swabs as needed. *(Zucker, p. 90)*

39.

D. Children are unable to understand death until the preadolescent period—the time when children become more concerned with other people. *(Model Curriculum, p.194)*

40.

C. The home care aide must respect the wishes of the family and follow the instructions of the care plans. *(Model Curriculum, p. 196)*

41.

A. Hearing is the last sense to go. Compassionate words and gentle touch will be reassuring to the dying patient. *(Zucker, p. 93)*

42.

B. The death rattle is a type of breathing that occurs as death approaches but the patient is still alive. *(Zucker, p. 93)*

43.

C. Mouth care is important for comfort and needs to be done often to remove crusty secretions. *(Zucker, p. 93)*

44.

C. Patients may deny death when talking about the future and avoid talking about their illnesses. *(Model Curriculum, p.195)*

45.

B. Honesty is very important, as is good listening. *(Zucker, p. 91)*

46.

D. The home care aide can help to change the patient's position. *(Zucker, p. 90)*

47.

A. An unwillingness to accept one's condition is called denial. *(Model Curriculum, p. 195)*

48.

C. Breathing may become irregular and stop for periods of time. *(Zucker, p. 93)*

49.

B. Care of the body after death is called postmortem care. *(Zucker, p. 94)*

50.

A. Keep the body flat on its back (supine), straightening the arms and legs. *(Zucker, p. 94)*

51.

B. Close the eyes, but do not press on the eyeballs. *(Zucker, p. 94)*

52.

B. If possible, place the dentures in the mouth to maintain the normal facial shape of the person. *(Zucker, p. 94)*

53.

B. Dying people have the same needs as the living, and avoidance of pain is a basic human need. *(Zucker, pp. 35, 89)*

54.

A. Hospice treats the patient and family as a unit of care. *(Zucker, p. 91)*

55.

C. The circulation slows as death approaches, and the arms and legs may feel cold and look ashen. *(Zucker, p. 93)*

56.

A. As the time of death nears, services or prayer rituals may be held at the bedside, and privacy will be requested. *(Zucker, p. 93)*

57.

B. Some caregivers wish to attend the patient's funeral. It gives them a formal chance to say goodbye. Examine your own feelings, and do what you feel is best. *(Zucker, p. 94)*

58.

B. Not everyone will experience every step in the dying process. *(Zucker, p. 89)*

59.

B. The needs of the dying and the living are the same: to spend time with family and friends. *(Zucker, p. 89)*

60.

C. The dying (and the living) have a need for some way to pass the time. These are just some examples of recreation. *(Zucker, p. 89)*

Practical Knowledge and Skills in Home Management

6 Infection Control

chapter objectives

Upon completion of Chapter 6, the student is responsible for the following:

➤ Differentiate among microorganisms, pathogens, and non-pathogens.

➤ Identify conditions necessary for microorganisms to grow and spread.

➤ Describe concepts of *clean* and *dirty*.

➤ Describe procedures for sterilization of equipment in the home.

➤ Define procedure for and importance of handwashing.

➤ Define standard precautions.

➤ Identify types of isolation and their uses.

➤ Define regulated medical waste.

DIRECTIONS
Each of the questions or incomplete statements below is followed by four suggested answers or completions. Select **one answer** that is best in each case.

1. Standard precautions are guidelines to be used:
   A. in caring for patients with AIDS only
   B. in caring for patients who are incontinent
   C. in caring for any patient
   D. only in the hospital setting

2. The most important way to prevent the spread of infection is to:
   A. wear gloves
   B. wear gowns
   C. wash hands
   D. wear masks

3. Standard precautions include:
   A. washing your hands in bleach water
   B. wearing sterile gloves at all times
   C. washing hands effectively
   D. isolating patients

4. Supplies to be used in patient care in the home should be kept:
   A. among things used by other family members
   B. in a clean area designated for the supplies
   C. in the kitchen cabinet
   D. in the car of the home care aide

5. To protect themselves from the spread of microorganisms when assisting patients with a productive cough, home care aides should:
   A. wear a mask and gown
   B. wear gloves
   C. wear goggles
   D. all of the above

6. Which of the following helps germs to multiply?
   A. moisture
   B. light
   C. temperatures below 40 degrees
   D. boiling water

7. Which of the following is one of the standard precautions?
   A. safety
   B. privacy
   C. dignity
   D. wearing gloves

8. If you think the person in your care is not infected, you:
   A. must follow standard precautions
   B. don't have to wear gloves
   C. don't have to change gloves between tasks
   D. don't have to handle linens carefully

9. You are wearing a gown while repositioning a patient with open sores. If the gown is not soiled:
   A. you should still discard it or bag it and send it to be washed
   B. you may use it while caring for another patient
   C. you should fold it and save it for use when caring for the same patient again
   D. you may use it at your home

10. Microorganisms that cause disease and infection are called:
    A. nonpathogens
    B. pathogens
    C. vehicles
    D. dirty

11. Clean areas of the patient's house may not contain:
    A. food
    B. dishes
    C. waste
    D. patient care supplies

12. Handwashing must be done before and after:
   A. food preparation for patient
   B. assisting patient with mouth care
   C. washing patient's dishes
   D. all of the above

13. A common type of microorganism that causes disease is a:
   A. bacterium
   B. leukocyte
   C. fomite
   D. host

14. What are pathogens?
   A. very small living organisms that can only be seen with a microscope
   B. disease-causing microorganisms
   C. medications that are used to treat disease
   D. toxic substances

15. Most bacteria grow best at:
   A. body temperature
   B. temperatures higher than body temperature
   C. temperatures cooler than body temperature
   D. temperatures below freezing

16. Pathogens are most likely to grow under which of the following conditions?
   A. sterile
   B. moist and dark
   C. dry and bright
   D. low temperatures

17. What should you do first when applying a gown?
   A. tie the strings at the neck
   B. tie the strings at the waist
   C. make sure it completely covers all of your clothing
   D. overlap the back of the gown

18. Pathogens use human tissue as their food and give off waste products called:
   A. bacteria
   B. toxins
   C. viruses
   D. organisms

19. A type of bacteria that lives in the colon where it helps to digest food is called:
   A. *Staphylococcus aureus*
   B. *Escherichia coli*
   C. infectious
   D. phagocyte

20. Bacteria that leave their normal environment and enter another part of the human body may cause:
   A. infection
   B. healing
   C. digestion
   D. urination

21. As a home care aide, you practice medical asepsis to:
   A. impress your supervisor
   B. impress your patients
   C. prevent the spread of pathogens
   D. enhance the spread of microorganisms

22. As a home care aide, you practice medical asepsis to prevent reinfection, cross-infection, and:
   A. breakage
   B. spilling
   C. spread of infection
   D. self-inoculation

23. Your patient develops the flu as a result of a visit from a church member who was sick. This is an example of:
   A. reinfection
   B. cross-infection
   C. self-inoculation
   D. vaccination

24. A cold is a disease that can be passed from person to person. These types of diseases are:
    A. self-infection
    B. asepsis
    C. communicable
    D. self-inoculation

25. A clean area of the patient's house would be:
    A. the toilet
    B. the basement sink
    C. the kitchen
    D. the bedside commode area

26. A dirty area of the patient's house would be:
    A. the kitchen
    B. the toilet
    C. the linen closet
    D. the laundry

27. Mrs. Tucker ate a hamburger that was contaminated with *E. coli.* This microorganism was spread by:
    A. animals
    B. clothing
    C. food
    D. air

28. The water faucet is always considered:
    A. clean
    B. dirty
    C. sterile
    D. aseptic

29. What is the first thing you should do when handwashing?
    A. work up a good lather with soap
    B. wash at least 2 inches above your wrists
    C. turn the faucet on with a paper towel
    D. use the nailbrush

30. If you place a paper towel near the sink and place your handwashing supplies on it, this area is considered:
    A. clean
    B. dirty
    C. sterile
    D. infected

31. While washing your hands and rinsing, you keep your fingertips pointed downward under running water. This is to:
    A. provide privacy
    B. prevent microorganisms from contaminating your arms
    C. keep the sink neat and clean
    D. make handwashing simpler

32. While handwashing, use a rotating and rubbing or friction motion for:
    A. 30 seconds
    B. 1 minute
    C. 3 minutes
    D. 5 minutes

33. After you have washed your hands, you notice that you have spilled water around the sink and countertop. You should:
    A. clean the area with another paper towel, then provide patient care
    B. clean the area with another paper towel, then wash hands again before providing patient care
    C. clean the area with disinfectant, then provide patient care
    D. clean the area with bleach, then provide patient care

34. The process of destroying as many harmful organisms as possible is called:
    A. sterilization
    B. vaccination
    C. disinfection
    D. isolation

35. Using an ammonia cleaner to clean up a urine spill is an example of:
    A. sterilization
    B. vaccination

C. disinfection

D. isolation

36. The process of killing all microorganisms is called:

A. sterilization

B. vaccination

C. disinfection

D. isolation

37. Bacteria that have formed hard shells around themselves as a defense are called:

A. viruses

B. yeast

C. spores

D. fungus

38. To kill spores, use the technique of:

A. sterilization

B. vaccination

C. disinfection

D. self-inoculation

39. Sterilization can be performed in the home by:

A. bleach

B. wet heat

C. pine cleaner

D. putting in the dishwasher

40. While performing wet-heat sterilization in the home, boil the object in water for:

A. 10 minutes

B. 15 minutes

C. 20 minutes

D. 25 minutes

41. The oven method of sterilization is an example of:

A. wet-heat sterilization

B. dry-heat sterilization

C. autoclave sterilization

D. baking sterilization

42. Disease-causing entities that are transmitted through contact with blood are known as:

A. contact pathogens

B. casual pathogens

C. blood-borne pathogens

D. intestinal pathogens

43. An example of a disease that is spread by blood-borne pathogens is:

A. AIDS

B. hepatitis A

C. tuberculosis

D. MRSA

44. Body fluids that are not considered contaminated include:

A. tears

B. sweat

C. saliva

D. urine

45. Isolation precautions that are initiated when a diagnosis of a specific pathogen is made are called:

A. universal precautions

B. transmission-based precautions

C. standard precautions

D. protective precautions

46. Equipment that is used to protect you from sources of contamination is known as:

A. protective barriers

B. work supplies

C. dirty equipment

D. used equipment

47. All of the following are examples of protective barriers except:

A. gloves

B. gowns

C. hair clasp

D. goggles

48. Gloves must be worn when in contact with:
    A. food
    B. sweat
    C. blood
    D. linens

49. Gowns or aprons are to be worn:
    A. for all patient care procedures
    B. when assisting the nurse with a Foley catheter change
    C. when taking out the trash
    D. when combing the patient's hair

50. The standard precautions and protective barriers to use when the patient is coughing excessively include:
    A. gloves
    B. gowns
    C. masks or face shields
    D. aprons

51. After washing your hands and applying your gloves before providing care, your patient asks, "Why do you wear those gloves? Am I unclean?" What is the appropriate response?
    A. "This is the standard of care for all the patients I see, and it is required."
    B. "Don't worry about it. You're fine."
    C. "Honey, you just never know what you'll be exposed to!"
    D. "You can't be too careful."

52. While emptying the pail for the bedside commode, you accidentally spill some of the urine on the bathroom tile floor. What should you do?
    A. Wait until you are finished with all your chores, then clean it up.
    B. While wearing gloves, wipe up the area, and then wipe with a solution of 1 part bleach to 10 parts water.
    C. Mop up the spill with a sponge mop.
    D. Spray the area with disinfectant.

53. How should you dispose of contaminated wound dressings?
    A. Throw them into the bathroom wastebasket.
    B. Burn them in the fireplace.
    C. Pour disinfectant over them and put in trash.
    D. Wrap the dressings in a plastic bag and double-bag before putting in the outside trash.

54. How often should soiled linen be washed?
    A. daily
    B. every other day
    C. when the regular laundry is washed
    D. every week

55. When you are caring for a patient with a highly contagious disease, your supervisor may instruct you on:
    A. disease precautions
    B. transmission-based precautions
    C. aseptic precautions
    D. universal precautions

56. When a patient is placed in basic isolation while at home, you should:
    A. let his or her dishes soak in the sink
    B. throw cleaning rags into the regular trash
    C. clean the urinal with soap and water
    D. use disposable dishes and cups, if available

57. Which of the following items is *not* contaminated?
    A. the outside of an isolation gown
    B. a wet mask
    C. the patient's towels in the bedside stand
    D. the pail in the bedside commode

58. Certain types of human waste are considered to be regulated medical waste. If you are

unaware of the regulations in your patient's community, you should:

A. burn all medical waste

B. flush all medical waste

C. contact your supervisor for details

D. all of the above

59. Which of the following is regulated medical waste?

A. a dressing that is soiled with blood

B. nasal mucus

C. sputum

D. emesis

60. Mr. Champ has a stiff beard, and you use a disposable razor to shave his face. The razor is:

A. human waste product

B. sharps

C. medical equipment

D. safe to reuse

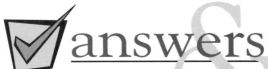

answers & rationales

1.

C. Standard precautions are actions that are taken on a routine basis for all patients. *(Zucker, p. 123)*

2.

C. Handwashing with soap and friction is the best way to prevent the transfer of microorganisms. *(Zucker, p. 119, 123)*

3.

C. Standard precautions are routine activities that are recommended to protect health care workers from contamination with blood and all body fluids except sweat. Washing your hands effectively is included in standard precautions. *(Zucker, p. 123)*

4.

B. Keep the environment and equipment clean with soap, water, and solutions that assist in keeping down bacterial growth. *(Zucker, p.118)*

5.

D. Masks, goggles, gowns, and gloves should be worn when the patient is coughing excessively. *(Zucker, p. 123)*

6.

A. Germs (microorganisms) grow well in damp places. *(Zucker, p. 116)*

7.

D. Gloves must be worn when contact is possible with blood and all body fluids except sweat. *(Zucker, p. 123)*

8.

A. Standard precautions are actions taken on a routine basis for all patients. *(Zucker, p. 123)*

9.

A. Gowns are for single-use purposes only. *(Zucker, p. 127)*

10.

B. Disease-producing microorganisms are called pathogens. *(Zucker, p. 116*

11.

C. No waste material is ever brought into a clean area of the house. *(Zucker, p. 118)*

12.

D. Handwashing must be done before and after each task and before and after direct patient contact. *(Zucker, p. 119)*

13.

A. Microorganisms can only be seen with a microscope, and they are very small living things, such as bacteria. A leukocyte is a white blood cell. A fomite is an inanimate object that may harbor microorganisms. The host is the individual who may be susceptible to disease from microorganisms. *(Zucker, p. 116)*

14.

B. Pathogens are microorganisms that cause disease. *(Zucker, p. 116)*

15.

A. Microorganisms such as bacteria need the correct temperature to live. Most cannot survive at high temperatures but live well at body temperature. *(Zucker, p. 117)*

16.

B. Pathogens, such as bacteria and viruses, grow best in darkness and in damp places. *(Zucker, p. 117)*

17.

C. Gowns should be long enough and large enough to cover clothing. *(Zucker, p. 127)*

18.

B. Toxins are the waste products of pathogens. Toxins are poisonous to the human body. *(Zucker, p. 116)*

19.

B. *E. coli* belongs in the human colon, where it helps to digest food. This is its normal living environment. *(Zucker, p. 116)*

20.

A. When bacteria, such as *E. coli,* leave the colon and enter the bladder, they can cause a urinary infection, for example. *(Zucker, p. 116)*

21.

C. Medical asepsis prevents the conditions that allow pathogens to live, multiply, and spread. *(Zucker, p. 116)*

22.

C. These are the main purposes for medical asepsis. *(Zucker, pp. 116–117)*

23.

B. Infection by a new or different type of microorganism from a visitor or member of the health care team is called cross-infection. *(Zucker, p. 117)*

24.

C. Communicable diseases are spread from one person to another. *(Zucker, p. 117)*

25.

C. A clean area of the house is one that is not contaminated by harmful microorganisms. *(Zucker, p. 118)*

26.

B. A dirty area of the house is one that is contaminated by harmful microorganisms. *(Zucker, p. 118)*

27.

C. Microorganisms are in many places and spread in various ways, in this case by food (hamburger). *(Zucker, p. 118)*

28.

B. The water faucet is always considered to be contaminated with pathogens. *(Zucker, p. 118)*

29.

C. Use paper towels to turn the faucet on and off. *(Zucker, p. 119)*

30.

A. By placing a paper towel near the sink (a clean area) and placing your clean equipment and supplies on it, you have designated this as your clean area. *(Zucker, p. 119)*

31.

B. Holding your hands downward prevents backflow over unwashed skin. *(Zucker, p. 119)*

32.

B. This amount of friction over 1 minute provides ample time to thoroughly clean all areas of the hand. *(Zucker, p. 120)*

33.

B. Of all these choices, you must wash your hands again after cleaning the sink and *before* providing patient care. This water spilled around the sink is considered contaminated. *(Zucker, p. 119)*

34.

C. Disinfection is the process of destroying most disease-causing organisms, as well as slowing down the growth and activity of the organisms that cannot be destroyed. *(Zucker, p. 121)*

35.

C. Disinfection removes as many harmful organisms as possible, and ammonia is a disinfectant. *(Zucker, p. 121)*

36.

A. Sterilization is the process of destroying all microorganisms, including spores, in a certain area. *(Zucker, p. 121)*

37.

C. Spores are bacteria that have formed hard shells around themselves for protection. *(Zucker, p. 121)*

38.

A. Spores can be destroyed only by sterilization, and some can even live in boiling water. *(Zucker, p. 121)*

39.

B. Wet-heat sterilization can be used in the home. *(Zucker, p. 121)*

40.

C. The contents of the pot of boiling water should be boiled undisturbed and covered for 20 minutes. *(Zucker, p.121)*

41.

B. Placing dressings in a pie tin in a 350°F oven for one hour is a form of dry-heat sterilization. *(Zucker, p. 122)*

42.

C. Diseases spread through exposure to blood and body fluids are called blood-borne pathogens. *(Zucker, p. 122)*

43.

A. AIDS is spread via human immunodeficiency virus, a blood-borne pathogen. *(Zucker, p. 123)*

44.

B. Standard precautions cover health care workers when exposed to all body fluids except sweat. *(Zucker, p. 123)*

45.

B. Transmission-based precautions are added to the plan of care when a definite diagnosis is made. *(Zucker, p. 124)*

46.

A. Protective barriers protect you from splashes, spills, droplets, or other sources of contamination. *(Zucker, p. 124)*

47.

C. Protective barriers are gloves, gowns, aprons, masks, face shields, and goggles. *(Zucker, p. 124)*

48.

C. Gloves must be worn when contact is possible with blood, all body fluids except sweat, skin that has breaks in it, and all mucous membranes. *(Zucker, p. 124)*

49.

B. Gowns or aprons must be worn during procedures or situations in which there may be exposure to blood, body fluids (except sweat), draining wounds, or mucous membranes. *(Zucker, p. 123)*

50.

C. Masks, face shields, or goggles must be worn when the patient is coughing excessively. *(Zucker, p. 123)*

51.

A. Gloves are to be worn whenever exposure to body fluids (except sweat) may occur. This is the new standard of care for all patients. *(Zucker, p. 123)*

52.

B. This is the procedure for cleaning a spill of body waste. *(Zucker, p. 124)*

53.

D. Double-bagging dressings protects you, the environment, and the people who handle the bags. Be sure the trash goes into a covered container. *(Zucker, p. 125)*

54.

A. Wash soiled linen each day. Keep soiled linen separate from the regular laundry, and handle with disposable gloves. *(Zucker, p. 126)*

55.

B. Additional precautions may need to be taken in caring for a patient with a highly contagious disease. Transmission-based precautions include contact precautions, droplet precautions, and airborne precautions. Your supervisor will give you specific instructions. *(Zucker, p. 126)*

56.

D. If available, use disposable dishes and cups; wash dishes separately in hot water and soap. Do not let dishes soak in the sink; cleaning rags should be disposed in plastic bags; the urinal should be cleaned thoroughly with disinfectant. *(Zucker, p. 127)*

57.

C. Each of the other items *is* contaminated. Patient care items stored in a clean location are not contaminated. *(Zucker, p. 128)*

58.

C. If you and your patient are not aware of the local regulations, your supervisor will be able to obtain the details. *(Zucker, p. 128)*

59.

A. Regulated medical waste is defined as blood, blood products, sharp medical instruments, and dressings contaminated with body fluids. *(Zucker, pp. 128–129)*

60.

B. Sharps should be disposed of in a metal container immediately after use. *(Zucker, p. 129)*

7 Clean, Safe, and Healthy Environment

chapter objectives

Upon completion of Chapter 7, the student is responsible for the following:

➤ Describe homemaking.

➤ Identify basic household cleaning tasks.

➤ Identify home safety issues and fire prevention and protection.

➤ Describe how to make equipment in the home.

DIRECTIONS Each of the questions or incomplete statements below is followed by four suggested answers or completions. Select **one answer** that is best in each case.

1. Before performing any procedure, the home care aide must first:
   A. provide privacy
   B. lower the bed rail
   C. explain the procedure
   D. gather supplies

2. All of the following will prevent falls except:
   A. locking the wheelchair
   B. dangling before transfer
   C. spills on the floor
   D. securing the bed rails

3. Oxygen therapy precautions include all of the following except:
   A. monitoring the amount of oxygen in the tank
   B. allowing the patient to smoke
   C. checking the oxygen tubing for kinks
   D. removing electrical appliances

4. Fire safety includes all of the following except:
   A. a fire escape plan
   B. teaching the patient safety precautions
   C. defective smoke detectors
   D. fire extinguishers on each level of the home

5. Safety precautions to follow in using electrical appliances include all of the following except:
   A. never overloading the circuits
   B. monitoring the floor for spills and debris
   C. inserting electrical plugs with wet hands
   D. replacing defective electrical cords

6. Poison precautions include all of the following except:
   A. keeping poisons out of the reach of children

   B. separating different people's medications in the same home
   C. unlabeled bottles
   D. good observations

7. Elderly patients are at risk for burns because they:
   A. may be overmedicated
   B. may be disoriented
   C. may be slow to feel hot temperatures
   D. may not follow smoking safety

8. Oxygen is considered a medication. Before assisting a patient with oxygen therapy, you should:
   A. take a class in oxygen use
   B. ask the patient how to change the reading
   C. call your supervisor
   D. call the equipment company

9. Who orders oxygen therapy?
   A. respiratory therapist
   B. registered nurse
   C. patient's family
   D. physician

10. Your patient has COPD and receives oxygen at 2 liters/minute by nasal cannula. As he is walking from the bedroom to the bathroom, he becomes short of breath and asks you to turn up his oxygen. The appropriate response should be:
    A. "How far do you want it turned up?"
    B. "I'm not allowed to adjust the oxygen. Rest for a moment, and you may feel well enough to adjust it yourself."
    C. "You'll have to wait until the nurse comes by."
    D. "Call the doctor."

11. Your patient is receiving oxygen therapy. She informs you that her oxygen canister is getting low. What should you do?
    A. Call the equipment company for immediate refill.
    B. Call the physician for more orders.
    C. Call the nurse care manager.
    D. Tell the patient to rest more.

12. An oxygen generator is delivered to your patient's home while you are there. The delivery person sets up the equipment but does not teach the patient how to use it. You should:
    A. report this to your supervisor
    B. turn on the machine
    C. call the doctor
    D. call the equipment company

13. Oxygen is delivered to the patient by all of the following except:
    A. a concentrator
    B. a vacuum canister
    C. a tank
    D. a liquid oxygen system

14. Oxygen precautions include reducing exposure to static electricity. Avoid all of the following except:
    A. cotton bedclothes
    B. television
    C. combing a patient's hair while he or she is receiving oxygen
    D. wool blankets

15. Your patient is receiving oxygen therapy via concentrator. Observe all of the following electrical safety precautions while providing care except:
    A. Do not use electric shavers.
    B. Do not use hair dryers.
    C. Do not use a microwave.
    D. Do not use heating pads.

16. Signs that a patient is receiving too much oxygen include all of the following except:
    A. rapid breathing
    B. sleepiness or difficulty waking up
    C. headache
    D. difficulty speaking

17. Signs that a patient is receiving too little oxygen include all of the following except:
    A. blue fingernails and/or lips
    B. confusion
    C. rapid speech
    D. tiredness

18. More accidents occur in the home than in any other place. This is due to:
    A. careful attention to detail
    B. ignorance of the potential hazards that exist in homes
    C. more elderly people being at home
    D. children playing in the home

19. Phone numbers that should be kept near the telephone for safety in your patient's home include all of the following except:
    A. police
    B. rescue squad
    C. poison control
    D. plumber

20. You note several scatter rugs around your patient's home and consider the patient to be at risk for falls. You should:
    A. remove all scatter rugs while the patient is sleeping
    B. discuss the safety hazard that scatter rugs are and ask the patient for permission to remove them
    C. tape down the edges of the scatter rugs
    D. call the doctor

21. Under the kitchen sink, you notice a spray bottle labeled "Bleach and Water." You should:

    A. use it to clean up spills of body waste

    B. spray soiled linens with this solution

    C. not use this solution

    D. clean the toilets with this solution

22. Your patient's two-year-old grandson spends the day with his grandparents. You should:

    A. insist that he be sent to day care

    B. keep the patient's bedroom door closed

    C. keep all poisonous substances in a high place behind locked doors

    D. provide your patient's care only when the grandson is asleep

23. Because temperature sensation becomes less accurate as we age, you should protect your patient from:

    A. falls

    B. tripping

    C. burns

    D. chemicals

24. Your patient lives in an old house that has few electrical outlets. You notice that the outlets are overloaded. You should:

    A. unplug anything that is not in use

    B. notify your supervisor

    C. request installation of additional outlets

    D. all of the above

25. Because your patient's bedroom has one electrical outlet, he has run an extension cord in from the living room and under the rugs in the hallway. Safety concerns involve:

    A. chemical spills

    B. electrical safety

    C. oxygen precautions

    D. width of the doorway

26. If you are uncomfortable in a house with cigarette smoke, you should:

    A. ask the people to put out their cigarettes

    B. ask the people to smoke outside

    C. discuss this with your supervisor

    D. ask for air filter machines to be placed in the home

27. When your patient is finished smoking, you should:

    A. empty the ashes into a plastic bag

    B. wet the ashes and then dispose of them

    C. empty the ashes into the plastic wastebasket

    D. empty the ashes into an old margarine dish

28. Mr. Thomas needs your assistance to get him ready for bed each evening. His wife gives him a sleeping pill each evening. Mr. Thomas requests your assistance with smoking. You should:

    A. provide him with the cigarette and sit with him

    B. tell him that he should not smoke at this time

    C. clean the bathroom while he smokes

    D. tell Mr. Thomas, "It's time you learned how to stop smoking."

29. While you are preparing fried bacon for your patient for breakfast, the oil catches on fire. You should extinguish it:

    A. with water

    B. with oil

    C. with baking soda

    D. by throwing the grease outside

30. Kitchen safety concerns in caring for the elderly include:

    A. not leaving cooking pots unattended

    B. deadbolts on doors

    C. outlet covers

    D. B and C

31. Mrs. Grace has some weakness in her legs, but she prefers to take a shower on a shower seat during your visits. You should:

    A. insist that she take a bed bath

    B. be sure that there is a secure bathmat on the floor

C. lift her into and out of the tub

D. give her privacy while waiting outside the door while she showers

32. Mrs. Brown has stacks of newspapers in a corner of her kitchen that are very old. You should:

A. take them outside and burn them

B. use them to wrap leftovers

C. arrange for them to be given to a recycling facility

D. move them to the basement

33. The necessary elements for a fire include all of the following except:

A. heat source

B. fuel

C. baking soda

D. oxygen

34. Which of the following is a fire safety concern?

A. There are no working smoke detectors.

B. There are fire extinguishers in the house.

C. The house is on one level with wide doors.

D. The patient is ambulatory.

35. In case of fire in your patient's home, your first action should be to:

A. seal off the fire

B. get your patient out of the house

C. call the fire department

D. go to a neighbor's house

36. Your patient forgets that he has taken his medication and takes more of it. This happens on a regular basis. This is considered to be:

A. normal

B. poisoning

C. negligence

D. acceptable as long as he does not get sick

37. You fear that Mr. Thomas has drunk some bleach that was sitting on the kitchen counter. He has dementia and was unaware that he was drinking bleach. You should:

A. induce vomiting

B. call the poison control center

C. call the doctor

D. make him drink milk

38. Your patient is receiving oxygen therapy. Upon completion of the bath, you may not rub the patient with:

A. baby lotion

B. aloe vera lotion

C. oil

D. baby powder

39. Mixing cleaning products will:

A. enhance the cleaning power

B. be more cost effective

C. potentially cause a chemical reaction that will hurt you

D. make your job go faster

40. When repairing electrical equipment in the patient's home:

A. unplug it

B. call your supervisor

C. open all electrical equipment with a knife

D. none of the above

41. Dusting is a homemaking task that home care aides may perform. In homes where people are particularly sensitive to dust, you may:

A. dust only once every two weeks

B. dust only once a week

C. have to dust often

D. not dust at all to avoid stirring up the dust

42. Dishes are more sanitary if:

A. baked in the oven

B. dried with a clean cloth

C. soaked

D. sprayed

43. The care plan for your patient includes kitchen cleaning. This would include all of the following except:
    A. wiping out the refrigerator on a regular basis
    B. wiping up the stove with soap and water
    C. wiping areas around drawer handles and door pulls
    D. wiping small appliances with soap and water while connected

44. A safety check in the bathroom would include all of the following except:
    A. grab bars in the shower or tub
    B. scatter rugs on the floor
    C. good lighting
    D. adequate ventilation

45. Equipment needed to clean the toilet includes all of the following except:
    A. bleach
    B. toilet bowl cleaner
    C. toilet bowl brush
    D. rag or sponge

46. Before washing, clothes should be sorted by:
    A. color
    B. fabric
    C. degree of dirt
    D. all of the above

47. A good time to vacuum the rugs and carpet in the patient's home is:
    A. while the patient is napping
    B. while the patient's family is sleeping
    C. when it is convenient for the patient and family
    D. immediately upon arrival at the patient's home

48. To minimize pests and bugs in your patient's home, you should:
    A. leave garbage uncovered
    B. leave trash inside the home until pickup
    C. put food away in closed containers
    D. clean up crumbs once a week

49. Cleaning to be done in the patient's home should be:
    A. acceptable and approved by the patient and family
    B. determined by the home care aide
    C. determined by the nursing supervisor
    D. avoided to ease your task load

50. The basic kinds of cleaning products include all of the following except:
    A. all-purpose cleaning agents
    B. soaps and detergents
    C. cleansers
    D. whatever the home care aide needs

51. All-purpose cleaning agents are useful for general housecleaning and may be used on all of the following surfaces except:
    A. countertops
    B. laundry
    C. walls
    D. floors

52. Soaps and detergents are used to clean all of the following except:
    A. baseboards
    B. laundry
    C. dishes
    D. bath

53. Specialty cleaners are used for special tasks and surfaces, such as:
    A. glass
    B. metal
    C. ovens
    D. all of the above

54. All of the following items are not permitted to be in dishwashers except:
    A. handpainted dishes
    B. stainless steel forks, knives, and spoons

C. fine glassware

D. electrical appliances

55. Basic mending tasks include all of the following except:

A. sewing on buttons

B. repairing ripped seams

C. making a dress

D. patching

56. Correct body mechanics in doing home maintenance tasks include all of the following except:

A. bend the knees

B. lift from the floor

C. keep shoulders up

D. stand as erect as possible

57. Which of the following should never be mixed together?

A. fabric softener and water

B. ammonia and chlorine bleach

C. ammonia and water

D. soap and starch

58. Housekeeping tasks that are done weekly include:

A. cleaning out the refrigerator

B. emptying bathroom wastebaskets

C. washing dishes

D. making beds

59. Lice can infest which part of the body?

A. head

B. hands

C. feet

D. all of the above

60. Mrs. Jones has a bright-colored housecoat that she wears when out of bed. It should be washed in which water temperature?

A. hot

B. warm

C. cold

D. dry-cleaned

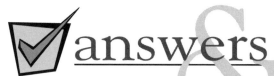

answers & rationales

1.

C. The patient has a right to know what you will be doing. *(Zucker, p. 5)*

2.

C. Removing spills promptly will help to prevent falls. *(Zucker, p. 148)*

3.

B. Oxygen precautions include no smoking. *(Zucker, p. 154)*

4.

C. A defective smoke detector is useless to detect smoke and fire. *(Zucker, p. 152)*

5.

A. Using wet hands to insert an electrical plug can result in an electrical burn or shock. *(Zucker, p. 150)*

6.

C. Do not assist a patient with a medication from an unlabeled container. *(Zucker, p. 318)*

7.

C. A normal aging change is decreased response to temperature changes, decreasing the ability to feel heat. *(Zucker, p. 54)*

8.

C. Your supervisor will tell you specific duties to assist with oxygen therapy. *(Zucker, p. 319)*

9.

D. Oxygen is prescribed by the physician. *(Zucker, p. 322)*

10.

B. Oxygen is considered a medication, and home care aides are not allowed to adjust the reading. At this time, resting may help him to catch his breath. *(Zucker, p. 322)*

11.

A. The equipment company is responsible for refilling the tank. *(Zucker, p. 322)*

12.

A. The equipment company is responsible for servicing the equipment and teaching the patient and family how to use it. If this does not occur, report it to your supervisor. *(Zucker, p. 322)*

13.

B. While the tank may look like a vacuum cleaner canister, the delivery systems are concentrators, tanks, and liquid oxygen. *(Zucker, p. 322)*

14.

B. Television poses no harm from static electricity to the patient who is receiving oxygen. *(Zucker, p. 320)*

15.

C. Small electric appliances used by or on the patient may spark and pose a fire hazard while the patient is receiving oxygen. The microwave poses no immediate safety risk to the patient. *(Zucker, p. 324)*

16.

A. Too much oxygen may be evidenced by slow, shallow breathing. *(Zucker, p. 324)*

17.

C. Too little oxygen would induce tiredness, not rapid speech, as well as irritability, anxiety, and/or restlessness. *(Zucker, p. 324)*

18.

B. Most people are unaware of the potential hazards that exist in homes. In addition, people are often careless and do not have safety inspections in homes as in commercial facilities. *(Zucker, p. 148)*

19.

D. Phone numbers should also include the fire department. *(Zucker, p. 149)*

20.

B. Respect the patient's home as his or her own. Discuss this with the patient before making these kinds of changes, although the rugs should be removed. *(Zucker, p. 148)*

21.

C. If a container does not have a proper label, do not use the contents. *(Zucker, p. 149)*

22.

C. Small children are at especially high risk of exposure to poisonous substances that are improperly stored. *(Zucker, p. 149)*

23.

C. Your patient is more susceptible to burns as a result of decrease in temperature sensation. *(Zucker, p. 149)*

24.

B. Overloaded outlets are a safety hazard in the home. Notify your supervisor so that he or she can assist the patient to correct this. *(Zucker, p. 150)*

25.

B. Do not put electrical cords under rugs. They may get frayed and can start a fire. *(Zucker, p. 150)*

26.

C. This is best discussed with your supervisor. If the patient is permitted to have smoking in his home, you may be asked to tolerate it. *(Zucker, p. 150)*

27.

B. When you empty ashtrays, be sure that the contents are cool. *(Zucker, p. 150)*

28.

B. A patient who has been given a sedative should not smoke. *(Zucker, p. 150)*

29.

C. Baking soda smothers the fire, which is the best way to extinguish a grease fire. (This also occurs with a chemical-type fire extinguisher.) *(Zucker, p. 150)*

30.

A. Do not leave cooking pots unattended. *(Zucker, p. 150–151)*

31.

B. Slippery floors are a significant safety problem in bathrooms. *(Zucker, p. 151)*

32.

C. Do not keep piles and piles of newspaper; arrange them for recycling. They are a fire hazard. *(Zucker, p. 151)*

33.

C. Baking soda smothers fire. *(Zucker, p. 150)*

34.

A. Smoke detectors are an important fire safety measure. *(Zucker, p. 152)*

35.

B. Get your patient to safety; then you may proceed with the other tasks. *(Zucker, p. 152)*

36.

B. Forgetting when they took their medications and taking additional doses of medication is considered poisoning. So is taking one medication when they should have taken another one. *(Zucker, p. 153)*

37.

B. The poison control center will know the exact antidote for ingestion of bleach. *(Zucker, p. 154)*

38.

C. Oil, alcohol, and talcum powder should not be used to rub the patient while oxygen is running. *(Zucker, p. 154)*

39.

C. Chemical reactions may hurt you and/or the surface you are cleaning. Do not mix cleaning products unless you have been instructed to do so. *(Zucker, p. 133)*

40.

A. Remove the equipment from its power source. Even though the equipment may be off, the electricity is live as long as its plugged in. *(Zucker, p. 134)*

41.

C. Dusting is done to prevent the spread of bacteria. Dusting often reduces the spread of microorganisms for people who are sensitive to dust. *(Zucker, p. 134)*

42.

B. Dry dishes with a clean cloth. *(Zucker, p. 134)*

43.

D. This can be done after the appliances have been disconnected from the wall outlet. *(Zucker, p. 135)*

44.

B. Scatter rugs are a falls hazard anywhere in the home. Rugs in the bathroom should have nonskid backing on tile floors. *(Zucker, p. 135)*

45.

A. You should not mix toilet bowl cleaner with any other cleanser. *(Zucker, p. 135)*

46.

D. Dark items should be separate from light colors, delicate fabrics separate from denim, and filthy jeans separate from underwear, for example. *(Zucker, p. 136)*

47.

C. Be sure the noise of the vacuum cleaner does not disturb the patient or family. *(Zucker, p. 137)*

48.

C. This prevents pests and bugs from exploring the patient's home, especially the kitchen. *(Zucker, p. 137)*

49.

A. Only cleaning that is acceptable to and approved by patients and their families should be done. *(Model Curriculum, p. 212)*

50.

D. Specialty cleaners are included in the basic kinds of cleaning products. *(Model Curriculum, p. 213)*

51.

B. Laundry should be cleaned by using laundry soap or detergent. *(Model Curriculum, p. 213)*

52.

A. All-purpose cleaning agents clean baseboards. *(Model Curriculum, p. 213)*

53.

D. Specialty cleaners address the specific needs of the task or surface. *(Model Curriculum, p. 213)*

54.

B. The silverware is safe in the dishwasher. Each of the other items is unsafe. *(Model Curriculum, p. 215)*

55.

C. Making a dress involves more than basic mending tasks. *(Model Curriculum, p. 217)*

56.

B. Lifting from the floor puts great strain on your lower back and is not good body mechanics. *(Model Curriculum, p. 222)*

57.

B. Ammonia and chlorine bleach, when mixed together, form a dangerous gas. *(Model Curriculum, p. 225)*

58.

A. The other tasks should be done daily. *(Model Curriculum, p. 234–235)*

59.

A. Lice can infest the head and other hairy parts of the body, resulting in severe itching. *(Model Curriculum, p. 239)*

60.

C. Cold is used for brightly colored and non-color-fast fabrics. *(Model Curriculum, p. 242)*

8 Nutrition and Fluids

chapter objectives

Upon completion of Chapter 8, the student is responsible for the following:

➤ Describe basic nutrition.

➤ Describe how to plan for, shop for, and serve a meal.

➤ Describe how to feed patients.

DIRECTIONS

Each of the questions or incomplete statements below is followed by four suggested answers or completions. Select **one answer** that is best in each case.

1. Nutrients are best defined as:
   A. food groups
   B. vitamins
   C. building blocks for the body's cells
   D. food substances for repair, maintenance, and growth of new cells

2. Nutrients include:
   A. carbohydrates
   B. iodine
   C. water
   D. all of the above

3. A well-balanced diet is one that provides:
   A. some food from each of the four food groups
   B. the prescribed amounts of servings of food listed on the food pyramid
   C. the proper amount of complete and incomplete proteins
   D. enough calories to produce heat for body function

4. Allergic reactions to food include:
   A. skin irritations
   B. swelling of the mouth and tongue
   C. difficulty breathing
   D. all of the above

5. A therapeutic diet is one that:
   A. is designed for a specific medical problem
   B. decreases or eliminates the use of salt
   C. provides for calorie reduction for weight loss
   D. provides for ethnic and religious preferences in food

6. The type of nutrient that builds and renews body tissues is:
   A. carbohydrates
   B. proteins
   C. fats
   D. vitamins

7. The recommended number of servings from the bread, cereal, rice, and pasta group a day for an adult is:
   A. 1 to 2
   B. 2 to 3
   C. 2 to 4
   D. 6 to 11

8. The recommended number of servings from the meat, poultry, fish, dry beans, eggs, and nuts group a day for an adult is:
   A. 1 to 2
   B. 2 to 3
   C. 2 to 4
   D. 6 to 11

9. The major differences in the diets of children and older adults is that:
   A. children need more protein and calories but older adults need more of other nutrients
   B. children need more carbohydrates and calories but older adults need more protein
   C. children need more fat and carbohydrates but older adults need more minerals
   D. children need more complete proteins and older adults need more incomplete proteins

10. The recommended number of servings of vegetables a day is:
    A. 1 to 2
    B. 2 to 3
    C. 3 to 5
    D. 6 to 11

11. The nutrient that builds and renews hemoglobin is:
    A. vitamin C
    B. carbohydrates
    C. iron
    D. iodine

12. A vitamin that is not stored in the body but is vital in helping the cells work together is:
    A. phosphorus
    B. iodine
    C. niacin
    D. ascorbic acid

13. Orange juice is an excellent source of:
    A. vitamin A
    B. vitamin B
    C. vitamin C
    D. vitamin D

14. An important nutrient to keep a person who is losing weight from losing muscle mass is:
    A. fat
    B. carbohydrates
    C. proteins
    D. minerals

15. A nutrient that is found in some table salt that is responsible for maintaining a healthy thyroid gland is:
    A. phosphorus
    B. iodine
    C. niacin
    D. ascorbic acid

16. Patients who are receiving radiation therapy may experience constipation, nausea, vomiting, and appetite loss. Change in their diet should include:
    A. an increase in red meat
    B. a decrease in fatty foods
    C. an increase in the intake of sugar and sweets
    D. all of the above

17. One way to help improve the appetite of a patient who is receiving radiation therapy or chemotherapy is to have the patient:
    A. eat small, frequent meals
    B. drink adequate amounts of cool, clear liquids
    C. use plastic utensils instead of metal ones
    D. all of the above

18. A patient on a low-residue diet should avoid:
    A. raw, fresh fruits and vegetables
    B. fried food, sauces, gravies, and ice cream
    C. canned vegetables, luncheon meat, and cheeses
    D. all of the above

19. To lower the patient's cholesterol, the doctor may recommend:
    A. poultry, fish, and red meat
    B. a limited amount of dairy food and fats
    C. no alcoholic beverages
    D. all of the above

20. A diabetic patient's diet must be followed very closely and restrict:
    A. alcoholic beverages
    B. high-sugar foods
    C. foods with corn syrup or honey
    D. all of the above

21. A patient on a low-salt diet should avoid:
    A. luncheon meats
    B. regular canned vegetables
    C. adding salt at the table
    D. all of the above

22. Patients on a mechanical soft diet could have:
    A. chopped or pureed food
    B. sauces and gravies
    C. ice cream and jello
    D. all of the above

23. When feeding a patient, you should remember:
    A. to allow the patient to do as much as possible for himself or herself
    B. that the patient may be resentful, so be friendly and natural
    C. to feed foods separately rather than mixed together
    D. all of the above

24. Safety factors to consider in feeding a patient include:
    A. when offering a glass or cup, touching it to the lips first
    B. not rushing the patient through the meal
    C. offering only small amounts
    D. all of the above

25. If a patient starts having difficulty swallowing food during a meal, you should:
    A. grind or mash up the food
    B. offer smaller bites
    C. notify your supervisor immediately
    D. all of the above

26. When assisting a patient to eat at the table, you should:
    A. keep the glass or cup of liquid out of the patient's reach
    B. place hot and cold food in separate bowls
    C. sit beside the patient
    D. all of the above

27. A major safety factor to remember in feeding a patient is:
    A. the temperature of the food
    B. not to offer a spoonful until the patient asks for it
    C. the patient's ethnic or religious preferences
    D. all of the above

28. To be sure a patient can swallow the current meal, you should:
    A. place the food as far back on the tongue as possible

B. give a very small amount of each food
    C. use a spoon instead of a fork
    D. all of the above

29. When feeding a patient, you could make meals more pleasant by:
    A. arranging the food in a clean, attractive manner
    B. offering a variety of foods
    C. protecting the patient's clothes without making an issue of it
    D. all of the above

30. In feeding a child, a major concern is:
    A. to offer only foods the child has eaten before
    B. to use small bowls
    C. to observe the child for acceptance of the diet
    D. All of the above

31. If feeding is the responsibility of the homemaker or home health aide, infants should be fed as often as:
    A. every 30 to 45 minutes
    B. every 3 to 4 hours
    C. identified by their family
    D. they demand to be fed

32. Observations of the pediatric patient for his acceptance of a diet include:
    A. the amount of gas following a feeding
    B. crying between meals
    C. diarrhea or constipation
    D. all of the above

33. When helping a mother as she breast-feeds, you should be aware that:
    A. the baby will alternate and feed from one breast at each feeding
    B. the mother will need to restrict her intake of fluids
    C. some medications and caffeine will pass to the baby
    D. all of the above

34. A breast-fed baby will:
    A. nurse 7 to 10 times a day during the first few months
    B. be affected by the mother's diet
    C. need to suck usually 6 to 8 minutes at each breast
    D. all of the above

35. Fluid intake for the mother who is breast-feeding should:
    A. be at least 6 to 8 glasses of water a day
    B. not contain caffeine
    C. not contain alcohol
    D. all of the above

36. If an infant is to be bottle-fed, you should:
    A. put the formula in bottles that are sterilized
    B. use the formula that you are most familiar with
    C. add cereal supplemental feeding at least twice a day
    D. all of the above

37. When feeding an infant, you must always:
    A. check the temperature of the formula
    B. prop the baby in bed or in the infant seat on its side to be fed, not on its back
    C. use a concentrated liquid formula
    D. all of the above

38. When feeding, ways to keep an infant from vomiting include:
    A. holding the bottle so that the nipple is full of formula and the baby does not suck air
    B. burping the baby after every two ounces of formula
    C. Not using formula that has been out of the refrigerator more than two hours
    D. all of the above

39. A frequent cause of diarrhea in a baby is:
    A. too much formula without cereal
    B. bacteria passed to the baby from the care-givers who have not washed their hands

    C. lack of appetite
    D. all of the above

40. If an infant is experiencing diarrhea, you should:
    A. notify your supervisor immediately
    B. increase the amount of liquids the infant takes orally
    C. tell the mother to change her diet
    D. all of the above

41. The normal 24-hour fluid intake for an average healthy adult is about:
    A. 3 1/2 quarts of fluid
    B. 6 to 8 quarts of fluid
    C. 10 to 12 pints of fluid
    D. 1 1/2 to 2 gallons of fluid

42. If the body is in a state of fluid balance, it is:
    A. maintaining an intake of more fluid than is lost
    B. eliminating as much fluid per day as is taken in
    C. maintaining a fluid output slightly more than is taken in
    D. normally excreting fluid from the body in urine and prespiration

43. The smallest amount of fluid that can be lost and result in death is:
    A. 10 percent
    B. 15 percent
    C. 20 percent
    D. 25 percent

44. Fluid imbalance is best described as:
    A. the amount of fluid drunk exceeds urinary output
    B. the amount of urinary output exceeds fluids taken into the body
    C. the amount of intake and output are not equal
    D. the inability of the patient to urinate adequately

45. For a patient who has a disease that may affect the body's fluid balance, the doctor may order:
    A. a water pill
    B. intake and output records
    C. forcing of fluids
    D. restriction of fluids

46. The term that best describes the condition that occurs when fluid loss exceeds intake is:
    A. fluid imbalance
    B. edema
    C. dehydration
    D. excretion

47. The term that best describes the condition that occurs when the body retains fluid in the tissue is:
    A. fluid imbalance
    B. edema
    C. cellulitis
    D. hydration

48. Fluids can be lost from the body through:
    A. the urine
    B. the intestinal tract
    C. the skin
    D. all of the above

49. Fluids can be lost from the body through:
    A. the lungs
    B. bowel movements
    C. emesis
    D. all of the above

50. If the patient is on force fluids, it is best for you to:
    A. offer liquids without being asked
    B. provide different types of liquids
    C. offer liquids in divided amounts
    D. all of the above

51. If the patient is on restricted fluids, you should:
    A. discourage the patient from drinking except when absolutely necessary
    B. encourage the patient to suck on ice chips
    C. offer liquids in divided amounts
    D. all of the above

52. Which of the following can influence the fluid balance in a person's body?
    A. the amount of exercise
    B. the weather
    C. medication
    D. all of the above

53. Another term for emesis is:
    A. excretus
    B. edema
    C. vomitus
    D. secretions

54. Making sure that the patient is adequately nourished and hydrated is critical because:
    A. it is your legal responsibility
    B. many illnesses can result from poor nutrition
    C. the kidneys can tolerate a fluid imbalance for only a short period of time
    D. intake and output are a nursing responsibility

55. Which of the following questions about the dietary needs of older adults is true?
    A. As a person grows older, digestion improves as food passes through the small intestine.
    B. Older people are able to better absorb and use nutrients.
    C. The intestinal muscle tone of the older adult decreases, resulting in constipation.
    D. Older adults need a high fat intake to maintain a feeling of warmth.

56. Important considerations in planning a menu for your patient include all of the following except:
   A. preparing many different kinds of foods
   B. preparing mild-tasting food
   C. preparing the food with familiar shapes
   D. choosing different types of texture within each meal served

57. Which of the following foods is a high source of vitamins?
   A. chicken
   B. wheat bread
   C. eggs
   D. water

58. Which of the following is a consideration in preparing a kosher meal for a Jewish patient?
   A. Au gratin potatoes and chicken are appropriate for dinner.
   B. Knives used to cut chicken are washed separately from knives used to cut cheese.
   C. Vegetables are served at only one meal each day.
   D. all of the above

59. When purchasing food for your patient, remember to:
   A. write down how much money you were given
   B. write down how much money you spent
   C. write down the amount of change you brought back
   D. all of the above

60. When buying foods that are high in protein, you can reduce the cost by:
   A. using red meat cuts
   B. using fillers such as bread crumbs or pasta to make a meat dish serve more
   C. use very tender cuts of meat for the elderly patient
   D. use beans and peas in limited quantity

61. Considerations for the home care aide feeding a patient include all of the following except:
   A. encouraging patients to feed themselves as much as possible
   B. mixing foods together to maximize taste
   C. recording intake and output
   D. standing next to the patient

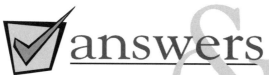

answers & rationales

1.

D. Nutrients come from many sources, such as foods and supplements. Other options are incorrect because, although vitamins are a type of nutrient, they are not the only type. Protein is considered the major building block for new cells and tissue. *(Zucker, p. 162)*

2.

D. All of these nutrients are needed by the body for it to function well. *(Zucker, pp. 163–165)*

3.

B. If you eat the correct number of servings from each food group, you will get the correct amount of each nutrient. *(Zucker, p. 162)*

4.

D. These are all symptoms of food allergies. The home care aide must observe for such reactions. *(Zucker, p. 167)*

5.

A. Therapeutic diets are ordered by the doctor to limit or increase the amounts of selected nutrients for a specific illness or problem. All patients' diets should provide for ethnic and religious food preferences. Low-salt and calorie reduction are both examples of therapeutic diets. *(Zucker, p. 172)*

6.

B. Carbohydrates provide energy for body activities; fats provide work energy and heat energy to maintain the body's temperature; vitamins are necessary for specific body functions. *(Zucker, p. 163)*

7.

D. This food group is found at the base of the pyramid, forming the foundation for the rest of the groups. Recommendations for the most servings are found at the bottom of the pyramid. *(Zucker, p. 163)*

8.

B. This food group is on the third tier of the food pyramid, and the recommendation is for fewer servings higher up the pyramid. *(Zucker, p. 163)*

9.

A. Dietary requirements are different at different stages of life. Because children are active, growing, and developing, they need more protein and calories than older people. *(Zucker, p. 162)*

10.

C. Vegetables are on the second tier of the pyramid and it is recommended that your have the second most number of servings per day from this group. *(Zucker, p. 163)*

11.

C. Iron is used by the body to carry oxygen from the lungs to the cells, in the form of hemoglobin. *(Zucker, p. 164)*

12.

D. Vitamin C acts as a cement between the body cells and helps them to carry out their special functions. Phosphorus, iodine, and niacin have other specific functions in the body. *(Zucker, p. 165)*

13.

C. Fresh, raw citrus fruits and their juices are sources of vitamin C. These include oranges, grapefruit, cantaloupe, and strawberries. *(Zucker, p. 165)*

14.

C. Protein is needed to build and renew body tissues, including muscles. Cutting back on fat and carbohydrates can help to decrease weight without decreasing muscle mass. *(Zucker, p. 163)*

15.

B. The thyroid gland needs iodine to control the rate at which foods are oxidized by the cells. None of the other choices are nutrients used by the thyroid gland. *(Zucker, p. 164)*

16.

B. Decreasing the intake of red meats, sweets, and fried or fatty foods will help to decrease nausea and decrease the intake of empty calories. *(Zucker, p. 172)*

17.

D. All of these measures may help to improve the appetite of a patient who is receiving radiation or chemotherapy. *(Zucker, p. 172)*

18.

A. Whole-grain products and uncooked fruits and vegetables contain high bulk, which stimulates the lower digestive tract. A low-residue diet eliminates foods that are high in bulk, so the lower digestive tract is spared excessive activity. *(Zucker, p. 173)*

19.

B. Foods containing animal fat such as eggs, milk, cheese, and meats are high in cholesterol. Poultry and fish have a lower fat content than other meats. Alcoholic beverages do not directly affect cholesterol levels. *(Zucker, p. 173)*

20.

D. Diabetic diets are designed to balance carbohydrates, proteins, and fats. Intake of high-sugar foods, alcohol, and carbonated beverages will increase the patient's blood sugar. *(Zucker, p. 173)*

21.

D. All of these choices contain salt or hidden sodium, which is to be avoided by patients on a low-salt diet. *(Zucker, p. 173)*

22.

D. Patients on this type of diet can have the same foods as on a normal diet, but chopped or strained. *(Zucker, p. 173)*

23.

D. Promote independence by allowing the patient to do for himself, put the patient at ease in the situation of being fed, and feed foods the way they are naturally eaten, not mixed together. *(Zucker, pp. 174–175)*

24.

D. The patient will be less likely to spill or choke if he or she knows that the glass or cup is at the mouth. Rushing can cause choking, as can giving the patient too large of a bite of food. *(Zucker, pp. 174–175)*

25.

C. The risk of choking is great when a patient has difficulty swallowing. A sudden onset of difficulty in swallowing could indicate a major medical problem. *(Zucker, p. 175)*

26.

C. When you sit down at the table with the patient, you are making the meal natural and social. You do not appear to be rushing when you sit down. *(Zucker, p. 174)*

27.

A. If a food is hot, tell the patient and then offer him or her a small amount to prevent burning the patient's mouth. Patients may not want to ask for every spoonful of food, and ethnic and religious preferences are not major safety issues during feeding. *(Zucker, p. 175)*

28.

B. If a patient will have difficulty swallowing, it is best to find out with a very small amount of food so that the patient does not choke or aspirate. *(Zucker, p. 175)*

29.

D. All of these actions help to make the patient's meal more pleasant. *(Zucker, pp. 174–175)*

30.

C. Careful observation will help determine any further dietary modifications. *(Zucker, p. 76)*

31.

C. Infants' feeding schedules vary greatly. Some are fed on-demand rather than on a specific hour schedule. Support the family as they follow what the physician has prescribed. *(Zucker, p. 76)*

32.

D. If you notice that a child has a great deal of gas following a meal, cries a great deal, has diarrhea or is constipated, or refuses food on a regular basis, report this to your supervisor immediately. *(Zucker, p. 76)*

33.

C. It is generally advised to avoid these medications and caffeine while nursing. Fluids should be increased by a nursing mother. The baby should nurse from each breast during every feeding. *(Zucker, p. 77)*

34.

D. All of these things are true of a breast-fed baby. *(Zucker, pp. 77–78)*

35.

D. Nursing mothers should avoid alcohol and caffeine, as it will enter the breast milk and affect the baby. Nursing mothers need to drink at least 6 to 8 glasses of water a day to help produce breast milk. *(Zucker, pp. 77–78)*

36.

A. Bottles are sterilized to destroy bacteria that might cause illness. The physician will determine when cereal should be fed to the infant and will prescribe the appropriate formula for the infant. *(Zucker, p. 78)*

37.

A. Check the temperature of the liquid in the bottle before giving it to the baby to prevent burns. Do not ever prop a bottle; rather, hold the baby when you feed him or her a bottle. Use the formula prescribed by the physician. *(Zucker, p. 80)*

38.

D. Choices A and B keep the baby from ingesting too much air, which may cause vomiting. Choice C helps to prevent feeding the child spoiled formula. *(Zucker, pp. 80–81)*

39.

B. Hand washing prevents the spread of bacteria from stool to the baby. Lack of appetite and formula do not cause diarrhea. *(Zucker, p. 82)*

40.

A. Diarrhea in infants can be a very serious problem, causing dehydration, so the supervisor should be made aware immediately. It is not within your role to increase the amount of liquids the infant takes or tell the mother to change her diet. *(Zucker, p. 82)*

41.

A. Choices A, B, and D are all more fluid than the average adult takes in during a 24-hour period. *(Zucker, p. 295)*

42.

B. Fluid balance is the relationship of intake fluid with excreted fluid output. When more fluid is taken in than is lost or more fluid is lost than taken in, a fluid imbalance exists. *(Zucker, p. 295)*

43.

C. Losing only one-fifth of the body's fluid will result in death. *(Zucker, p. 295)*

44.

C. Fluid imbalance exists when intake and output are unequal. It does not matter whether output exceeds intake or intake exceeds output; both result in fluid imbalance. *(Zucker, p. 295)*

45.

B. Accurate records of intake and output indicate how the fluid balance system of the body is functioning. Water pills and fluid restriction would not be appropriate for a patient with dehydration; forcing fluids would not be appropriate for a patient with edema. *(Zucker, p. 296)*

46.

C. Fluid imbalance may occur when intake exceeds output or when output exceeds intake. Dehydration occurs when output exceeds intake. *(Zucker, p. 296)*

47.

B. The type of fluid imbalance that causes swelling and fluid to be held in body tissues is edema. Cellulitis is a type of inflammation. Hydration refers to the amount of fluid in the body. *(Zucker, p. 296)*

48.

D. All of these are ways in which the body eliminates fluids. *(Zucker, p. 295)*

49.

D. Fluid leaves the body as water vapor in exhaled air, in bowel movements, particularly if they are soft or loose, and in vomit. *(Zucker, p. 295)*

50.

D. All of these actions will help to increase the patient's fluid intake. *(Zucker, p. 303)*

51.

C. When a patient is on fluid restriction, the amount he or she may have is divided up to last throughout the day. You should offer liquids in appropriate amounts during the day. The patient may or may not be permitted to suck on ice chips; check with your supervisor about that. *(Zucker, p. 303)*

52.

D. Fluid can be lost during exercise. It can be lost as sweat during hot weather. Medications can cause fluid loss or retention. *(Zucker, p. 296)*

53.

C. Vomit and vomitus both refer to regurgitated food and fluid. *(Zucker, p. 295)*

54.

B. Observing and reporting nutritional and fluid status are very important. Serious illnesses and complications can be prevented or minimized if action is taken early. *(Zucker, pp. 172, 296)*

55.

C. This is a normal part of aging, and it takes longer for food to digest as we age. *(Zucker, p. 55)*

56.

B. A combination of flavors is important to taste. Serve strong-flavored foods as a spotlight, and keep milder-tasting foods as the background in a meal. *(Zucker, p. 166)*

57.

B. Grains are excellent sources of many vitamins. Meat, poultry, and dairy products are not. Water has no vitamin content. *(Zucker, pp. 164–165)*

58.

B. Utensils and equipment used for meat products are kept separately from those used for dairy products. Meat and dairy products may not be eaten at the same meal. *(Zucker, p. 167)*

59.

D. Under the guidance of your supervisor, document all of these items and be certain that the patient understands what you spent, on what, and how much change was returned. *(Zucker, p. 169)*

60.

B. This does make a meat dish go farther. Use poultry when it is cheaper than meat. Beans and peas can be substituted for higher-cost meats. *(Zucker, p. 169)*

61.

B. Feed the foods separately rather than mixed together. *(Zucker, p. 175)*

III

Practical Knowledge and Skills in Personal Care

9 Vital Signs

chapter objectives

Upon completion of Chapter 9, the student is responsible for the following:

➤ Define adult normal rates for vital signs.

➤ Measure and report oral, axillary, and rectal temperatures.

➤ Measure and report pulse rate and rhythm.

➤ Measure and report respiratory rate.

➤ Measure and report blood pressure.

➤ Define systolic and diastolic blood pressures.

DIRECTIONS
Each of the questions or incomplete statements below is followed by four suggested answers or completions. Select **one answer** that is best in each case.

1. Temperatures should be taken orally when the person is:
   A. on oxygen
   B. paralyzed
   C. alert and cooperative
   D. having trouble breathing

2. Which of the following is a normal oral temperature?
   A. 96.2 degrees
   B. 98.6 degrees
   C. 99.5 degrees
   D. 101.1 degrees

3. Which of the following respiration rates is normal for an adult?
   A. 70 breaths per minute
   B. 20 breaths per minute
   C. 10 breaths per minute
   D. 60 breaths per minute

4. A thermometer should be cleaned by:
   A. washing thoroughly in cool sudsy water, rinsing, and then repeating the wash and rinse
   B. washing in alcohol and then wiping dry with a cotton pad
   C. placing in a container of boiling water and then wiping with alcohol
   D. pouring boiling water over the thermometer and then wiping with alcohol

5. Which of the following is a normal reading for a rectal temperature?
   A. 98.0 degrees
   B. 99.6 degrees
   C. 97.8 degrees
   D. 96.6 degrees

6. Which of the following pulse readings is normal for an adult?
   A. 42 beats per minute
   B. 110 beats per minute
   C. 76 beats per minute
   D. 20 beats per minute

7. An oral temperature should not be taken if a patient:
   A. is short of breath or is having trouble breathing
   B. is over the age of 25
   C. is lying in bed
   D. has recently had rectal surgery

8. As a person gets older, blood pressure generally:
   A. tends to get lower
   B. stays the same as it was when the person was younger
   C. tends to rise
   D. tends to rise in males only

9. Why do you not use the thumb to take a person's radial pulse?
   A. The thumb has its own pulse, and you may count your pulse rate instead of the person's.
   B. The thumb is too big.
   C. The thumb gets in the way of your other fingers.
   D. Using your thumb causes you to press too hard.

10. Vital signs include all of the following except:
    A. pulse
    B. temperature
    C. weight
    D. respirations

11. In which of the following instances should you check the patient's vital signs?
    A. The patient is sleeping comfortably.
    B. The patient has been vomiting for two hours.
    C. The patient has just finished breakfast.
    D. The patient has had a bowel movement.

12. If the patient has recently had a cup of hot coffee:
    A. wait 10 minutes before taking his or her temperature
    B. take the patient's temperature and subtract 1 degree
    C. take the patient's temperature and record it
    D. wait 1 hour before taking his or her temperature

13. The apical pulse is located:
    A. on the arm
    B. on the leg
    C. on the chest
    D. on the neck

14. The instrument used to measure the apical pulse is the:
    A. stethoscope
    B. sphygmomanometer
    C. hand
    D. all of the above

15. The key element to accurate measure of a patient's respirations is to:
    A. count the respirations without the patient knowing it
    B. use a stethoscope
    C. wait until the patient is sleeping
    D. count the respirations first thing in the morning

16. For the most accurate assessment of the radial pulse of a patient, the pulse should be counted for:
    A. 10 seconds
    B. 15 seconds

C. 30 seconds
D. 60 seconds (one full minute)

17. The term "vital signs" refers to:
    A. temperature, pulse, and respiration
    B. temperature, pulse, respiration, and blood pressure
    C. blood pressure, pulse, and respiration
    D. blood pressure, temperature, and pulse

18. The balance between the heat produced by the body and heat lost by the body is measured as:
    A. pulse
    B. respiration
    C. temperature
    D. blood pressure

19. The rate at which the heart is beating is measured as:
    A. pulse
    B. respiration
    C. temperature
    D. blood pressure

20. The process of inhaling and exhaling is measured as:
    A. pulse
    B. respiration
    C. temperature
    D. blood pressure

21. The force of blood pushing against the walls of the arteries is measured as:
    A. pulse
    B. respiration
    C. temperature
    D. blood pressure

22. You should check the vital signs of your patient:
    A. if you observe any change in the patient
    B. if the patient falls
    C. when your supervisor instructs you to do so
    D. all of the above

23. Which piece of equipment do you use to measure temperature?
    A. thermometer
    B. stethoscope
    C. sphygmomanometer
    D. watch with a second hand

24. Which piece of equipment do you use to measure the radial pulse rate?
    A. thermometer
    B. stethoscope
    C. sphygmomanometer
    D. watch with a second hand

25. Which piece of equipment do you use to measure the respiratory rate?
    A. thermometer
    B. stethoscope
    C. sphygmomanometer
    D. watch with a second hand

26. Which piece of equipment is used to listen to blood pressure?
    A. thermometer
    B. stethoscope
    C. sphygmomanometer
    D. watch with a second hand

27. Which artery is used to measure the blood pressure?
    A. radial
    B. carotid
    C. brachial
    D. femoral

28. The systolic pressure is a measurement of:
    A. high blood pressure
    B. the heart contracting as it pumps the blood into the arteries
    C. the lower number
    D. stress

29. The diastolic pressure is a measure of:
    A. low blood pressure

B. the highest pressure
C. sleep
D. the heart relaxing between each contraction

30. The average normal blood pressure reading for adults is:
    A. 80/58
    B. below 120/80
    C. below 140/90
    D. 160/90

31. Before taking an axillary temperature, the home care aide should:
    A. lubricate the thermometer
    B. be sure to have a rectal thermometer
    C. dry the armpit if it is moist
    D. shave the armpit

32. What is the appropriate time frame for measurement of a rectal temperature?
    A. 3 minutes
    B. 7 minutes
    C. 8 minutes
    D. 9 minutes

33. When taking a rectal temperature, the home care aide should do all of the following except:
    A. lubricate the tip of the thermometer
    B. insert the thermometer 1/2 inch and hold it in place
    C. leave the patient unattended
    D. wear gloves

34. Respiration is best described as:
    A. one inhalation
    B. one exhalation
    C. one inhalation and one exhalation
    D. none of the above

35. Your patient is breathing very loudly and seems to be working hard to get his breath. This is called:
    A. normal respiration
    B. labored respiration

C. effort respiration

D. stress respiration

36. If the patient is breathing using only the upper part of the lungs, this is called:

A. stertorous respiration

B. abdominal respiration

C. shallow respiration

D. irregular respiration

37. The type of respiration that is very irregular and frequently occurs before death is called:

A. stertorous respiration

B. abdominal respiration

C. shallow respiration

D. Cheyne-Stokes respiration

38. The type of respiration in which the depth of breathing changes and the rate of the rise and fall of the chest is not steady is called:

A. stertorous respiration

B. abdominal respiration

C. shallow respiration

D. irregular respiration

39. You have just completed taking the patient's vital signs, and she asks you what they are. How should you respond?

A. "You don't need to worry about that."

B. "I'm only supposed to tell my supervisor."

C. "Sure! Here they are . . ."

D. "They're just fine."

40. The patient's normal blood pressure reading is 120/80. Today the reading is 90/60. What should you do?

A. Nothing. The patient just needs to move around some more.

B. Report this to your supervisor right away.

C. Get the patient out of bed and to the shower.

D. Tell the patient to get some more rest.

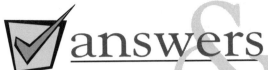

answers & rationales

1.

C. It is best for the patient to be alert and cooperative for you to measure oral temperature. *(Zucker p. 273)*

2.

B. The normal oral range of body temperatures is 97.6 to 99 degrees. *(Zucker p. 273)*

3.

C. Normally adults breathe at a rate of 16 to 20 times a minute. *(Zucker p. 272)*

4.

A. This is the actual procedure for cleaning a thermometer. Use cool water only. *(Zucker p. 277)*

5.

B. The normal range of rectal body temperature is 98.6 to 100 degrees. *(Zucker p. 273)*

6.

C. The average normal adult pulse rate is 60 to 80 regular beats per minute. *(Zucker p. 272)*

7.

A. Shortness of breath and trouble breathing may alter the oral temperature reading as well as distress the patient while the oral temperature is being obtained. *(Zucker p. 278)*

8.

C. A normal physiological change of aging is that blood pressure tends to rise. In adults over 40 years old, 160/90 or less is considered normal. *(Zucker p. 288)*

9.

A. Never use your thumb. Your thumb has its own pulse, and you may count it instead of the patient's. *(Zucker p. 283)*

10.

C. The term "vital signs" refers to body temperature, pulse rate, respiratory rate, and blood pressure, *not* weight. *(Zucker p. 271)*

11.

B. You should check vital signs if you observe any change in your patient or after a fall. *(Zucker p. 271)*

12.

A. Hot or cold liquids or smoking will alter the oral temperature reading. Wait 10 minutes before taking the oral temperature. *(Zucker p. 278)*

13.

C. The apical pulse is located and measured at the apex of the heart, just below the left nipple. *(Zucker p. 282)*

14.

A. A stethoscope is used to listen to the apical pulse. *(Zucker p. 282)*

15.

A. You want to count the natural breathing of the patient, which is best achieved when the patient does not know you are counting. *(Zucker p. 286)*

16.

D. Counting the pulse for one full minute is the most accurate measure. *(Zucker p. 283)*

17.

B. The term "vital signs" refers to blood pressure, pulse rate, respiratory rate, and temperature. *(Zucker p. 269)*

18.

C. This is the definition of temperature. *(Zucker p. 271)*

19.

A. This is the definition of pulse. *(Zucker p. 271)*

20.

B. This is the definition of respiration. *(Zucker p. 271)*

21.

D. This is the definition of blood pressure. *(Zucker p. 271)*

22.

D. Your supervisor will tell you when and how often to check your patient's vital signs on the basis of the patient's present condition, past history, and prognosis. *(Zucker p. 272)*

23.

A. The body temperature is measured with an instrument called a thermometer. *(Zucker p. 274)*

24.

D. The radial pulse rate is measured with the use of a watch with a second hand. *(Zucker p. 283)*

25.

D. The respiratory rate is measured with the use of a watch with a second hand. *(Zucker p. 287)*

26.

B. You will use a stethoscope to listen to the brachial pulse as you measure blood pressure. *(Zucker p. 289)*

27.

C. When you take a patient's blood pressure, you use a stethoscope to listen to the brachial pulse. *(Zucker p. 289)*

28.

B. The heart contracts as it pumps the blood into the arteries. When the heart is contracting the pressure is highest, and this pressure is the systolic pressure. *(Zucker p. 288)*

29.

D. As the heart relaxes between each contraction, the pressure goes down. When the heart is most relaxed, the pressure is lowest; this pressure is called the diastolic pressure. *(Zucker p. 288)*

30.

C. The average normal blood pressure for adults 18 to 50 years old should be below 140/90. *(Zucker p. 272)*

31.

C. If the axillary region is moist with perspiration, pat it dry with a towel. *(Zucker p. 280)*

32.

A. The home care aide should hold the thermometer in place for 3 minutes. *(Zucker p. 279)*

33.

C. Do not leave a patient with a rectal thermometer in the rectum, no matter what his or her condition. *(Zucker p. 279)*

34.

C. One respiration includes breathing in once and breathing out once. *(Zucker p. 286)*

35.

B. If the patient seems to be working hard to get his or her breath, it is called labored respiration. *(Zucker p. 286)*

36.

C. Shallow respiration is when the patient breathes using only the upper part of the lungs. *(Zucker p. 286)*

37.

D. This breathing begins slow and shallow; then the respiration becomes faster and deeper until it reaches a kind of peak; then it slows down and becomes shallow again and may even stop completely for a period of time. This frequently occurs before death. *(Zucker p. 286)*

38.

D. This is the description of irregular respiration. *(Zucker p. 286)*

39.

C. Especially in a person's home, you will be expected to share the vital sign readings with your patient. Please do so promptly. *(Zucker p. 272)*

40.

B. You should report changes from what is normal for each patient; in this case, the blood pressure is much lower than normal. *(Zucker p. 272)*

10 Elements of Body Function

chapter objectives

Upon completion of Chapter 10, the student is responsible for the following:

- ➤ Describe bed making.
- ➤ Define body mechanics.
- ➤ Identify the patient's level of ability.
- ➤ Describe bed positioning and bed mobility.
- ➤ Describe perineal care.
- ➤ Identify urinary drainage systems.
- ➤ Describe ostomy care.

DIRECTIONS
Each of the questions or incomplete statements below is followed by four suggested answers or completions. Select **one answer** that is best in each case.

1. Problems associated with dehydration include:
   A. skin breakdown
   B. weakness
   C. dry mouth and eyes
   D. all of the above

2. In caring for the bedbound patient who is experiencing incontinence, the home care aide should:
   A. provide frequent perineal care
   B. have the nurse insert a catheter
   C. always use adult diapers
   D. none of the above

3. Major considerations in the prevention of constipation include:
   A. hydration
   B. nutrition
   C. enemas
   D. A and B

4. Concerns that should be reported in caring for the patient with a urinary catheter include:
   A. leaking around the catheter
   B. fever or chills
   C. blood in the urine
   D. all of the above

5. In caring for the patient with a urinary catheter, the urinary collection bag should:
   A. be on the bed with the patient
   B. be above the level of the urinary bladder
   C. be below the level of the urinary bladder
   D. be on the floor

6. What action should the home care aide include when caring for the patient who is frequently incontinent?
   A. Provide perineal care following each incident.
   B. Monitor underpads frequently for wetness or soiling.
   C. Withhold fluids.
   D. A and B

7. All of the following stimulate bowel function except:
   A. fruits
   B. vegetables
   C. grains
   D. limited fluids

8. When placing the patient on the bedpan, the home care aide should perform the following activities except:
   A. have the patient raise hips and slide the bedpan under
   B. have the patient position the bedpan if able
   C. have the patient roll to one side, place the bedpan, and have the patient roll back
   D. grease the bedpan with lubricant

9. Which of the following is a good principle of body mechanics?
   A. Keep your knees locked.
   B. Keep the person a few inches away from your body.
   C. Place your feet about 12 inches apart with one foot slightly ahead of the other.
   D. Twist your upper body as you lift.

10. Wrinkles in the bed linen should be avoided because:
    A. they can cause the person to sweat
    B. they can cause skin irritations and bed-sores
    C. they cause extra wear on the sheets
    D. they can cause wear spots on the mattress

11. Which statement about the use of drawsheets is true?

A. Drawsheets are used only for moving people with contractures.

B. Drawsheets assist the home care aide in positioning a person in bed.

C. Drawsheets are used to absorb excess urine when a person is incontinent.

D. Drawsheets decrease the need to change linens.

12. As a home care aide, which of the following can you do to help a person who has breathing problems?

A. Take cigarettes away from a person every time he or she smokes.

B. Raise the head of the bed when the person is lying down.

C. Encourage the person not to take rapid, shallow breaths.

D. Tell the person to avoid taking deep breaths.

13. You are helping a patient walk to the living room. He is getting short of breath. You should:

A. let him stop and rest

B. encourage him to walk faster to the living room

C. leave him and call for help

D. encourage him to stay in his room in the future

14. A consistent rule to follow regarding when to change bed linens is to:

A. change the bottom sheet once a day

B. change all linens immediately if they are wet or contaminated

C. change the top sheet once a week

D. change only the drawsheet once a day

15. A home care aide can help female patients to avoid becoming incontinent by:

A. encouraging them to hold their urine a few minutes before they eliminate

B. washing the perineal area from front to back

C. giving fluids once a day

D. responding quickly to the patient's request to go to the bathroom or use a bedpan

16. Which one of the following is *not* something a home care aide should do to make sure a patient's digestive system works as well as possible?

A. Encourage exercise.

B. Allow enough time for eating.

C. Encourage patients to eat sweets.

D. Make sure patient has regular bowel movements.

17. Which of the following statements is *not* correct in providing perineal care for a person with a urinary catheter?

A. Make sure the drainage bag is attached to the bed and that it is higher than the person's bladder.

B. Always clean the perineum from front to back.

C. Make sure tubing is not kinked.

D. Make sure the drainage bag and tubing are not touching the floor.

18. A bed that remains empty for a while is called a:

A. closed bed

B. open bed

C. occupied bed

D. surgical bed

19. The type of bed that is made when the patient is able to get out of bed and move around is called a:

A. closed bed

B. open bed

C. occupied bed

D. surgical bed

20. The type of bed that is made while the patient is in the bed is called the:

A. closed bed

B. open bed

C. occupied bed

D. surgical bed

21. Wrinkles in the patient's bed are uncomfortable and may cause:
    A. constipation
    B. itching
    C. bedsores
    D. incontinence

22. Which of the following guidelines is appropriate for bed making?
    A. Use a pin to hold torn sheets together.
    B. The bottom sheet must be firm, smooth, and wrinkle free.
    C. Hold the linen closely against you when transporting it.
    D. Use a plastic garbage bag to protect the sheets.

23. Which is the first step in making an occupied bed?
    A. Loosen all the sheets around the bed.
    B. Ask the patient to turn onto his side.
    C. Remove the old bottom sheet from the bed.
    D. Change the pillowcase.

24. Mrs. Brooks has very sensitive sores on the tops of her shins and knees. To prevent the sheets from touching her toes, you could make a:
    A. foot board
    B. backrest
    C. bed table
    D. bed cradle

25. Mr. Burns had a CVA 6 years ago and has foot drop in his right foot. This condition may have been prevented with the use of:
    A. a bed cradle
    B. a walker
    C. a foot board
    D. foot soaks

26. Practicing good body mechanics will help to prevent:
    A. constipation
    B. back injury
    C. weight gain
    D. all of the above

27. To be certain that you are supporting your patient's center of gravity, support him:
    A. by holding his right arm
    B. at the waist
    C. by holding his left arm
    D. from behind

28. Helping your patient to move her buttocks out over her feet to get from a sitting to a standing position is evidence of which principle of body mechanics?
    A. base of support
    B. center of gravity
    C. balancing
    D. strongest muscles

29. Your body is properly aligned when:
    A. your back is straight
    B. your knees are straight
    C. your weight is on the strong foot
    D. you are 12 inches away from the patient

30. When you are moving along with your patient and you want to change direction, you should:
    A. turn with long, smooth steps
    B. turn your whole body without twisting your neck and back
    C. pivot on one foot
    D. all of the above

31. Your patient prefers to sleep and spend all his time on the couch. Since you cannot raise the couch, you must remember to:
    A. bend over the couch to reach all areas
    B. put your foot on a stool to relieve pressure in your back
    C. insist on a hospital bed
    D. have someone help with all care

32. The patient and family must know how to give care when you are not there. They learn best from:
    A. your example
    B. neighbors
    C. relatives
    D. books

33. A patient who is bedridden should have his position changed:
    A. at least every 2 hours
    B. when requested
    C. after meals
    D. when you have help

34. Arrangement of the patient's body in a straight line, with body parts placed in anatomical position, is known as:
    A. body mechanics
    B. functional
    C. body alignment
    D. center of gravity

35. A patient has had a stroke and is unable to move by himself. When changing his position, you note a pressure sore developing on his sacrum. This could delay:
    A. muscle tightness
    B. rehabilitation
    C. skin breakdown
    D. all of the above

36. Mrs. Smith has had a stroke and has a paralyzed right side. You should refer to her paralyzed right leg as:
    A. "the bad side"
    B. "the functional leg"
    C. "the involved leg"
    D. "the good side"

37. The patient has scooted down in the bed and needs to be moved up. She can stand briefly with assistance. You can reposition her up at the head of the bed by:

A. pulling on her arms to pull her up in bed
B. helping her to stand and move her buttocks up toward the head of the bed
C. lifting her up in bed
D. leaving her until help arrives

38. To reposition a patient with right-sided weakness, you will:
    A. position and support only functional parts of the body
    B. position and support all parts of the body
    C. position and support the legs
    D. position and support only nonfunctional parts of the body

39. To position a patient on his or her back, you should:
    A. place a large, fluffy pillow under the head
    B. tuck in the sheets snugly
    C. place the weak arm and elbow on a pillow higher than the heart
    D. put a washcloth in the uninvolved hand

40. After you have positioned a patient on his involved side, you should change his position:
    A. more frequently than when he is positioned on the uninvolved side
    B. at the same time intervals as when he is positioned on the uninvolved side
    C. less frequently than when he is positioned on the uninvolved side
    D. every 15 minutes

41. If a family member wishes to help you move the patient up in bed, you should:
    A. have the family member move the legs while you move the upper body
    B. have the family member move the upper body while you move the legs
    C. review the procedure with the family member before you move the patient
    D. hold the patient under the arms and pull upward

42. If a patient's body is correctly aligned in bed, the spine should be:
    A. twisted to relieve pressure
    B. slightly curved
    C. arched at the lower back
    D. straight

43. Shearing can be reduced by:
    A. lifting or rolling patients
    B. changing the patient's diet
    C. sliding patients whenever possible
    D. rubbing bony prominences

44. Bedridden patients are turned regularly to avoid:
    A. high blood pressure
    B. skin breakdown
    C. respiratory failure
    D. heart attack

45. In turning a patient, it is helpful if the patient:
    A. crosses his or her legs
    B. remains as stiff as possible
    C. is asleep
    D. holds onto the side rail in the direction in which he or she is turning

46. Which of the following statements about elimination frequency is true?
    A. Elimination frequency varies greatly from one person to another.
    B. Elimination frequency never varies, regardless of a patient's condition.
    C. Most people have bowel movements every 3 days.
    D. Most people need to urinate every 2 hours.

47. When a patient has to wear incontinence briefs, you should:
    A. wait for the patient to ask to be changed
    B. refer to the briefs as diapers
    C. urge the patient not to wet the bed
    D. report any perineal skin changes to your supervisor

48. An indwelling catheter is used to:
    A. help patients with diarrhea
    B. continuously remove urine from the bladder
    C. increase fluid output
    D. decrease fluid intake

49. Perineal care for the patient with a Foley catheter:
    A. can be eliminated until the catheter is removed
    B. should be done normally as if there were no catheter
    C. should include liberal amounts of talcum powder
    D. is done once a day in the morning

50. Condom catheters are:
    A. inserted at the urinary meatus
    B. changed at least every 24 hours
    C. replaced once or twice a month
    D. permanently attached to the patient

51. Which of the following statements about perineal care is true?
    A. It is important to encourage the patient to do his or her own perineal care.
    B. You should always do perineal care for the patient.
    C. Perineal care is done only when a patient is incontinent.
    D. Perineal care is not required for males.

52. Which of the following statements about incontinence is true?
    A. Only patients who are fully mobile should be allowed to eliminate in private.
    B. A patient will be able to control his or her elimination better if he or she is helped to the bathroom promptly.
    C. Patients in your care should be required to use the toilet on a regular schedule.
    D. Patients who have been in a nursing home in the past will not be embarrassed about needing help with elimination.

53. Weak and small muscle groups are located in the:
    A. thighs
    B. back
    C. hips
    D. shoulders and upper arms

54. An object is very heavy. You should not:
    A. pull it
    B. push it
    C. lift it
    D. roll it

55. You are going to move a patient up in bed. The bed should be:
    A. raised at the foot
    B. in the low horizontal position
    C. as flat as possible
    D. raised at the head

56. You are going to use a drawsheet or pull sheet to turn a patient. Grasp the sheet at the:
    A. shoulders and knees
    B. waist and knees
    C. shoulders and buttocks
    D. waist and shoulders

57. Mrs. Little is sitting in a chair while her bed is being made. The top linens are folded back so that she can get into bed. This is:
    A. an open bed
    B. a closed bed
    C. a surgical bed
    D. an occupied bed

58. Mrs. Cochran will be out of bed most of the day. The type of bed you should make is the:
    A. open bed
    B. closed bed
    C. surgical bed
    D. occupied bed

59. Plastic drawsheets do all of the following except:
    A. protect the bottom linens
    B. increase the risk of skin breakdown
    C. protect the mattress
    D. increase the patient's comfort

60. A colostomy is a surgical opening into the:
    A. ileum
    B. bladder
    C. large intestine
    D. stomach

61. The pink part of the colostomy that you see on the patient's abdomen is called the:
    A. mucous membrane
    B. stoma
    C. anus
    D. conduit

62. Which can be used to clean the skin around a stoma?
    A. hydrogen peroxide
    B. detergent
    C. soap and water
    D. alcohol

63. The gastrostomy is a surgical opening directly into the:
    A. esophagus
    B. nose
    C. stomach
    D. colon

64. A urine specimen that has no contamination by anything outside the patient's body is called a:
    A. midstream specimen
    B. clean-catch specimen
    C. 24-hour specimen
    D. catheter specimen

65. In assisting the patient to obtain a stool specimen, it is important to remember to:
    A. ask the patient not to urinate into the bedpan or put tissue in the bedpan
    B. have the patient have a bowel movement into the toilet
    C. take 1/2 cup of the stool specimen and put it into the specimen container
    D. rinse the specimen with water

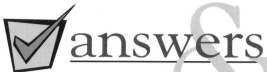

answers & rationales

1.

D. Lack of fluids and dehydration are significant risk factors associated with skin breakdown, patient weakness, and dry mouth and eyes and any mucous membrane. *(Zucker, pp. 295–296)*

2.

A. Perineal care will help to prevent infection for the bedbound patient. *(Zucker, pp. 226–227)*

3.

D. Normal bowel activity relies on adequate hydration and proper nutrition (e.g., fiber intake). *(Zucker, p. 55)*

4.

D. Leaking and blood in the urine should be reported to the supervisor, as well as fever or chills, which may be signs of infection. *(Zucker, p. 327)*

5.

C. The urinary collection bag should be attached to the bed frame (while the patient is in bed) lower than the patient's urinary bladder to facilitate drainage via gravity. *(Zucker, pp. 327–328)*

6.

D. Keeping the perineal area clean is essential to prevent skin breakdown. Checking the pads frequently to be sure they are dry also helps to protect the area from skin breakdown. *(Zucker, pp. 226–227)*

7.

D. Adequate amounts of fruits, vegetables, and grains, along with six to eight glasses of water daily, help to maintain normal bowel function. *(Zucker, 163)*

8.

D. The bed pan may be dusted with powder to prevent sticking, but using lubricant would be messy and uncomfortable for the patient. *(Zucker, pp. 223–224)*

9.

C. Placing your feet at least 12 inches apart provides a broad base of support and good balance. *(Zucker, pp. 178–179)*

10.

B. Keep linen wrinkle free and dry at all times to reduce the risk of skin breakdown. *(Zucker, p. 195–196)*

11.

B. For patients who cannot move themselves, a draw-sheet or pull sheet can help the home care aide move the patient in bed more easily. *(Zucker, pp. 182–183)*

12.

B. Raising the head of the bed may ease the breathing for the patient. *(Zucker, p. 189)*

13.

A. Permit the patient to rest. Once the shortness of breath stops, you may continue. *(Zucker, pp. 107–108)*

14.

B. Keep the bed dry and clean; change the linen when necessary. *(Zucker, p. 139)*

15.

D. Responding to the patient's request will help her to maintain her normal urinary schedule. *(Zucker, p. 222)*

16.

C. Regular activity, chewing and eating properly, and regular bowel movements assist the patient's digestion. *(Zucker, pp. 108–109)*

17.

A. The drainage bag must be lower than the patient's bladder to facilitate drainage. *(Zucker, pp. 226–227, 329)*

18.

A. The closed bed is usually made when it will remain empty for a while. It is made with a bedspread or only with a sheet and blanket. *(Zucker, p. 140)*

19.

B. The open bed is used when it will be occupied within a short period of time and the patient is able to get up and move around. *(Zucker, p. 140)*

20.

C. The occupied bed is made when the patient is not able or not permitted to get out of bed. *(Zucker, p. 144)*

21.

C. Home care aides should make beds with no wrinkles in the sheets because they are uncomfortable and can cause bedsores. *(Zucker, p. 138)*

22.

B. This makes the patient more comfortable and prevents skin breakdown. *(Zucker, p. 139)*

23.

A. Of the steps listed, this is the first you would perform. *(Zucker, pp. 145–147)*

24.

D. A bed cradle is used under the blankets and sheets and over the patient's legs so that the covers do not touch the skin. *(Zucker, p. 158)*

25.

C. A foot board is used to support the covers so that they do not touch the patient's toes and to provide a place where the patient can rest his foot. It helps to prevent foot drop. *(Zucker, pp. 158–159)*

26.

B. Body mechanics helps to protect your back and your job. *(Zucker, p. 177)*

27.

B. A person's center of gravity is located around the pelvic area. By supporting the patient at the waist level, you will have the greatest amount of control over the patient's movements. *(Zucker, p. 178)*

28.

C. The patient's center of gravity will be balanced over his or her base of support—this will help the patient to balance quite well and stand more easily. *(Zucker, p. 178)*

29.

A. Use good posture. Proper body alignment includes keeping the back straight, the knees bent, and weight evenly distributed on both feet. *(Zucker, p. 178)*

30.

B. Avoid twisting your back and neck; turn your whole body. *(Zucker, p. 178)*

31.

B. The same rules of body mechanics apply for situations in which you are unable to raise the bed area to a comfortable position for you. *(Zucker, p. 179)*

32.

A. By setting a good example, you will teach and will assist the patient and family in accepting their limitations and provide good care. *(Zucker, p. 180)*

33.

A. The position must be changed every 2 hours for comfort and to prevent skin breakdown. *(Zucker, p. 181)*

34.

C. This is the definition of body alignment or bed positioning. All of the patient's body parts are in their proper positions in relation to each other. *(Zucker, p. 182)*

35.

B. If a patient who is not properly positioned in bed develops a bedsore, it will have to heal before he or she can start exercises. *(Zucker, p. 182)*

36.

C. This is the side involved with treatment. There is nothing "bad" about that body part. *(Zucker, p. 182)*

37.

B. This is an excellent way to get her in the correct bed position, and she will have exercised her muscles, heart, balance, and coordination. *(Zucker, p. 183)*

38.

D. The rest of the body parts should be left free to move. *(Zucker, pp. 183–184)*

39.

C. This will assist with circulation and help extra fluid to drain from the limb. *(Zucker, pp. 183–184)*

40.

A. The patient's comfort is essential, and being positioned on the involved side may be painful. *(Zucker, p. 184)*

41.

C. The family member may not know how to do this procedure using good body mechanics. *(Zucker, p. 186)*

42.

D. Body alignment is the correct positioning of the patient's body, with the body and spine straight. *(Zucker, p. 182)*

43.

A. Lifting or rolling patients is the proper way to move and position patients and eliminate shearing. *(Zucker, p. 193)*

44.

B. Regular repositioning of bedridden patients will reduce the chance of skin breakdown. *(Zucker, pp. 181–182)*

45.

D. Expect the patient to do as much as possible. This task will also assist your efforts. *(Zucker, p. 181)*

46.

A. The bladder and the bowel respond to receptors that send messages to the brain. This varies for each person. *(Zucker, pp. 109–110)*

47.

D. Proper cleansing of the perineal area to decrease exposure to urine will decrease the risk of skin irritations. *(Zucker, pp. 226–227)*

48.

B. The indwelling catheter is used when a patient is unable to urinate naturally. *(Zucker, p. 327)*

49.

B. Keep the patient's perineal area clean. Even though he or she may not be urinating as usual, mucus and perspiration collect in the area. *(Zucker, p. 329)*

50.

B. This device should not be left on for more than 24 hours at a time and must be removed at least that often so that the penis may be washed and inspected. *(Zucker, pp. 331–332)*

51.

A. A great principle of care is to encourage patients to do as much for themselves as possible, especially with perineal care. *(Zucker, pp. 226–227)*

52.

B. Prompt trips to the bathroom decrease the number of episodes of incontinence. *(Zucker, pp. 195–196)*

53.

B. Generally, the muscles that flex (bend) the joints—your arms, shoulders, and legs—are the strongest, not those in your back. *(Zucker, pp. 178–179)*

54.

C. You should not lift a very heavy object. This puts great strain on your weaker back muscles. *(Zucker, p. 179)*

55.

C. This enables you to move the patient without resistance. *(Zucker, p. 185)*

56.

C. This distributes the weight evenly. *(Zucker, p. 186)*

57.

A. The open bed is made when the patient is able to get out of bed and move around. *(Zucker, pp. 140, 144)*

58.

B. The closed bed is made when it is expected to be empty for a while. *(Zucker, p. 140)*

59.

D. They decrease the patient's comfort because they may increase sweating. *(Zucker, p. 139)*

60.

C. This is a surgically created opening through the abdominal wall through which waste material (feces) is discharged. *(Zucker, p. 336)*

61.

B. The stoma is a surgically created opening and will look like a pink rosebud. *(Zucker, p. 336)*

62.

C. The entire ostomy area can be washed with soap and water on a washcloth, using a gentle circular motion. *(Zucker, p. 338)*

63.

C. The gastrostomy is a surgically created opening for the patient to receive part or all of his or her nourishment through this opening. *(Zucker, p. 339)*

64.

B. The term "clean-catch" refers to the fact that the urine is not contaminated by anything outside the patient's body. *(Zucker, p. 311)*

65.

A. It is important not to contaminate the desired specimen with other body fluids or foreign matter. *(Zucker, p. 315)*

11 Emergencies

chapter objectives

Upon completion of Chapter 11, the student is responsible for the following:

➤ Identify steps to take in an emergency.

➤ Describe how to dislodge a foreign body in the airway.

➤ Define first aid for controlling external bleeding.

➤ Define first aid for burns.

➤ Identify signs and symptoms of a heart attack.

➤ Define first aid for a victim of a heart attack.

DIRECTIONS
Each of the questions or incomplete statements below is followed by four suggested answers or completions. Select **one answer** that is best in each case.

1. A home care aide discovers a fire in the patient's home. The first action should be to:
   A. close the doors to the area where the fire is occurring
   B. move the patient to safety
   C. call the supervisor
   D. call the fire department

2. Mrs. Cochran is walking with the home care aide and begins to fall. The home care aide should:
   A. attempt to hold Mrs. Cochran upright until help arrives
   B. allow Mrs. Cochran to fall so that both of you won't be hurt
   C. gently lower Mrs. Cochran to the floor
   D. call for help

3. Upon arrival at your patient's home this morning, you find him on the floor. You should:
   A. sit the patient upright
   B. call the supervisor
   C. move all the patient's joints to check for fracture
   D. put the patient back in his bed

4. During an emergency in the home, the home care aide should:
   A. panic
   B. give commands to the patient's family
   C. run for help
   D. remain calm

5. After you have fixed Mr. Bell's breakfast, you return to his bedroom to find that he has fallen on the floor. What should you do?
   A. Stay with Mr. Bell and shout for help.
   B. Assist Mr. Bell to a chair and then call for help.

   C. Call for your nurse supervisor for immediate advice.
   D. Assist Mr. Bell back into bed.

6. Which procedure is used for a choking victim?
   A. CPR
   B. Heimlich maneuver
   C. blows on the back
   D. raising the arms upward

7. When you enter your patient's room, you check him and note that he is unconscious. What is your first response?
   A. check for breathing
   B. start CPR
   C. call your supervisor
   D. check for pulse

8. All of the following are emergency treatments for burns except:
   A. pressure
   B. ice pack
   C. cold water
   D. sterile dressings

9. You suspect that your patient is having a heart attack. You should do all of the following except:
   A. check for response
   B. give the patient an antacid
   C. check for breathing
   D. check for circulation

10. The food that most commonly causes an airway obstruction is:
    A. pudding
    B. soup
    C. meat
    D. juice

11. A patient who is choking will:
    A. say, "I am choking."
    B. clutch at his or her throat
    C. appear flushed
    D. take slow, deep breaths

12. The Heimlich maneuver is not effective if the patient is:
    A. pregnant
    B. lying down
    C. sitting
    D. standing

13. When performing the Heimlich maneuver on a patient who is standing, you should do all of the following except:
    A. stand behind the patient
    B. wrap your arms around the patient's waist
    C. place the thumb side of one fist on the abdomen between the navel and the sternum and grasp with the other hand
    D. press your fist and hand into the patient's abdomen with a quick, downward movement

14. Life-threatening situations include all of the following except:
    A. choking
    B. flu
    C. heart attack
    D. no pulse

15. Which of the following situations is a life-threatening emergency?
    A. Your patient's pulse decreases.
    B. Your patient refuses to eat.
    C. Your patient is in shock.
    D. Your patient is withdrawn.

16. The first action you should take upon discovering an emergency situation is to:
    A. file an incident report
    B. ask the patient's family what to do
    C. call or send for help
    D. begin CPR

17. What happens during myocardial infarction?
    A. damage to the heart muscle
    B. breathing stops owing to a blocked airway
    C. pulse and respiration increase rapidly
    D. the brain has a seizure

18. Your patient has no pulse. To restore circulation, you should use:
    A. the finger sweep
    B. chest compressions and mouth-to-mouth breathing
    C. the Heimlich maneuver
    D. mouth-to-mouth breathing only

19. If a choking victim is coughing forcibly, you should:
    A. immediately begin the Heimlich maneuver
    B. allow the coughing to continue
    C. use mouth-to-mouth breathing
    D. try to get the person to stop coughing

20. The finger sweep is used to:
    A. restore circulation
    B. reduce injury during a seizure
    C. clear the blocked airway of an unconscious person
    D. administer medications

21. If a patient is undergoing a seizure, it is essential to:
    A. restrain the patient
    B. protect the patient from infection
    C. hold his or her tongue down with your fingers
    D. protect the patient from physical injury

22. When a patient is having a seizure, you should:
    A. use restraints to limit the patient's movement
    B. tighten the patient's clothing
    C. place an object in the patient's mouth to prevent injury
    D. place a towel or blanket under the patient's head

23. Some patients know that they are going to have a seizure. This is called:
    A. a premonition
    B. an aura
    C. petit mal
    D. a vision

24. Your patient is having a seizure, and you note that her whole body is stiff, and she is jerking and unconscious. This type of seizure is:
    A. petit mal
    B. idiopathic
    C. grand mal
    D. progressive

25. Mr. Thomas is prone to seizures. Today, you note that he is sitting in his chair and appears to be daydreaming, but his eyes are rolled back and his lips are quivering. This type of seizure is:
    A. petit mal
    B. idiopathic
    C. grand mal
    D. progressive

26. While observing your patient have a seizure, actions you can take include:
    A. moving the patient to a bed
    B. opening the patient's mouth to insert a tongue depressor
    C. turning the patient's head to the side to promote drainage of saliva or vomitus
    D. All of the above

27. After your patient has a seizure, important actions you can take include:
    A. loosening restraints
    B. giving the patient milk to drink
    C. notifying the doctor
    D. assisting the patient with mouth care

28. What is the first action the home care aide can perform before assisting a patient with an obstructed airway?
    A. call the supervisor
    B. give five back blows
    C. ask the patient whether he or she is choking or able to speak
    D. perform a finger sweep

29. How many abdominal thrusts should the home care aide perform on a choking patient?
    A. 1 or 2 thrusts
    B. 3 or 4 thrusts
    C. 5 thrusts
    D. as many as needed until the object is expelled

30. Your patient appears to be choking with a complete airway obstruction. Your action should be to:
    A. perform CPR
    B. perform the Heimlich maneuver
    C. call your supervisor
    D. give five back blows

31. Which one of the following observations would tell the home care aide that her patient's airway is completely obstructed?
    A. The patient is making clear coughing sounds and his or her eyes are tearing.
    B. The patient is holding his or her neck and making no sound.
    C. The patient says, "I'm choking."
    D. The patient is vomiting.

32. Abdominal thrusts are best described as:
    A. applying pressure to the sternum
    B. applying inward and upward pressure rapidly to the middle to upper abdomen
    C. applying pressure to the chest
    D. applying pressure to the lower abdomen

33. All of the following methods are performed during the Heimlich maneuver except:
    A. standing behind the person
    B. wrapping your arms around the person's waist

C. making a fist and placing the thumb side into the abdomen

D. placing your arm around the person's chest

34. Which is an effective position for the home care aide to assist with an obstructed airway?

A. Stand behind the person.

B. Stand facing the person.

C. Stand to the left of the person.

D. Stand to the right of the person.

35. A sign of partial blockage when a patient is choking is:

A. snoring sounds

B. unable to speak

C. cool skin

D. fainting

36. In an emergency, common first aid practices would include:

A. moving the person from floor to bed

B. leave the person to get someone else to help

C. control bleeding

D. administer oxygen

37. As a home care aide, you may be required to perform artificial breathing. What personal protective equipment should you carry for your protection?

A. gloves

B. pocket face shield

C. gown

D. mask

38. You are caring for an 8-month-old infant who tries to swallow a marble, which becomes lodged in her airway. You should do all of the following except:

A. a blind finger sweep

B. calling out for help

C. delivering up to five back blows forcefully between the shoulder blades with the heel of one hand

D. providing up to five quick downward chest thrusts with two fingers

39. Timmy, a 6-year-old boy in your care, tried to swallow a whole hot dog, which lodged in his airway and caused complete airway obstruction. You should do all of the following except:

A. abdominal thrusts

B. call for help immediately

C. back blows

D. none of the above

40. When performing rescue breathing on an unconscious adult, you must:

A. give one breath every 3 seconds

B. give 10 to 12 breaths per minute

C. give 16 to 20 breaths per minute

D. give him or her something to drink

41. Rescue breathing for an infant or small child must be given:

A. every 3 seconds

B. every 5 seconds

C. every 10 seconds

D. only when medical help arrives

42. Excessive bleeding from a severe cut is called:

A. leukemia

B. shock

C. hemorrhage

D. menstruation

43. While you are assisting Mr. Smith with shaving with a disposable razor, he turns suddenly, and you accidentally cut him right on the jawbone. He begins to bleed. The blood vessels that were damaged are:

A. the arteries

B. the veins

C. the capillaries

D. large

44. Mrs. Thomas has arthritis and is using a rocking knife to cut an apple. She accidentally loses control of the knife, which causes a 1-inch cut across her forearm. It appears to be deep, and the blood is oozing out. The blood vessels that were damaged are:
    A. the arteries
    B. the veins
    C. the capillaries
    D. large

45. Your patient falls and badly breaks her leg— a compound fracture. Blood is spurting from the fractured area. The blood vessels that were damaged are:
    A. the arteries
    B. the veins
    C. the capillaries
    D. small

46. When treating external blood loss, you should do all of the following except:
    A. apply direct pressure over the wound with a clean cloth
    B. if possible, elevate the limb to decrease the blood supply
    C. apply a tourniquet
    D. remain with the person until help arrives

47. Severe blood loss can lead to:
    A. hypertension
    B. shock
    C. infection
    D. increased urine production

48. You suspect that your patient has accidentally drunk some kitchen cleaner, and he is now unconscious. You should:
    A. give him a glass of milk
    B. position him on his back.
    C. call for help and remain with him until help arrives
    D. induce vomiting

49. Poisoning by inhalation of chemicals and gases will cause reactions such as:
    A. vomiting
    B. increased appetite
    C. hyperactivity
    D. irritations of eyes, throat, and skin

50. On a pleasant summer morning, your patient decides to sit outside. Shortly, you hear him yell, "I've been stung!" and he has a large red mark on his neck. You should observe for other signs of allergic reaction except:
    A. difficulty breathing
    B. swelling
    C. appetite
    D. tingling in the area of the bite

51. Signs and symptoms of shock include all of the following except:
    A. the face is bright red
    B. the eyes are dull and the pupils are wide
    C. respirations are shallow, irregular, and labored
    D. the pulse is rapid and weak

52. Emergency treatment for shock will include:
    A. giving the person some bicarbonate of soda
    B. encouraging the person to sleep
    C. positioning the person with the head lower than the legs
    D. turning on a fan

53. Mr. Brown turned on the hot water in the bathroom and received a burn on his hand, which caused blistering. This is a:
    A. first-degree burn
    B. second-degree burn
    C. third-degree burn
    D. fourth-degree burn

54. Complications from burns include all of the following except:
    A. good body image
    B. infection

C. pain

D. shock

55. When providing emergency treatment for a first degree burn, you will:

   A. remove clothing stuck to the burned area

   B. put the body part in cool water if possible

   C. apply petroleum jelly

   D. put ice on the burn

56. Mr. Evans has a second-degree burn on his legs from boiling water spilled from the stove. Your emergency treatment would include all of the following except:

   A. not removing clothing stuck to the burned area

   B. dowsing with cool water

   C. covering the area with sterile or clean dry cloth or sheet

   D. wetting the dressing

57. Most heart attacks occur during:

   A. intense physical activity

   B. sex

C. sleep

D. eating

58. Classic symptoms of a heart attack include all of the following except:

   A. pain like a belt around the chest

   B. pulse rate slow

   C. color is pale

   D. wet clammy skin

59. Emergency treatment for heart attack includes all of the following except:

   A. calling for medical help

   B. giving the person some ginger ale to drink

   C. loosening clothing if it is tight

   D. providing rescue breathing if breathing has stopped

60. Signs and symptoms of a cerebrovascular accident (stroke) include all of the following except:

   A. full movement of all extremities

   B. headache

   C. change in consciousness

   D. difficulty with speech or vision

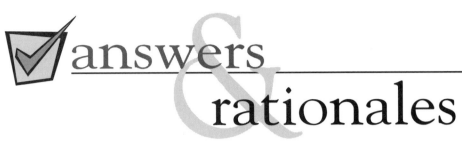

answers & rationales

1.

B. Get the patient out of the house. *(Zucker, p.152)*

2.

C. Know your capabilities; gently lower the patient to the floor. *(Zucker, pp. 240, 375–376)*

3.

B. Contact your supervisor when any unusual event occurs. *(Zucker, p. 27)*

4.

D. This will permit you to think, respond, and act appropriately. *(Zucker, p. 375)*

5.

C. Contact your supervisor when any unusual event occurs. *(Zucker, p. 27)*

6.

B. The Heimlich maneuver applies pressure to the upper abdomen to dislodge an obstruction by a foreign body in the airway. *(Zucker, p. 379)*

7.

C. Calling for help and guidance will greatly assist the patient *(Zucker, p. 375)*

8.

A. Pressure is not a treatment for burns. *(Zucker, p. 385–386)*

9.

B. Do not give the patient anything to eat or drink. *(Zucker, p. 388)*

10.

C. Larger pieces of food, such as meat, are a common cause for choking. *(Zucker, p. 377)*

11.

B. This is the universal sign for choking. *(Zucker, p. 378)*

12.

A. Do not use the Heimlich maneuver on the obese, pregnant women, infants, or small children. *(Zucker, p. 380)*

13.

D. Quick, upward thrusts should be given. *(Zucker, p. 379)*

14.

B. The flu is not life-threatening unless it progresses to respiratory distress. The other situations are imminently life-threatening. *(Zucker, p. 375)*

15.

C. The other situations may concern you but are not life-threatening. *(Zucker, p. 384)*

16.

C. Emergencies are situations that call for immediate action. Call or send for help. *(Zucker, p. 375)*

17.

A. Heart function and circulation stop because of damage to the heart muscle. *(Zucker, p. 386–387)*

18.

B. Chest compressions stimulate the heart to circulate the blood, and mouth-to-mouth breathing provides needed oxygen. (This is CPR.) *(Zucker, p. 387)*

19.

B. Do not interfere with the person if he or she is able to cough. *(Zucker, p. 378)*

20.

C. The finger sweep is used for removal of an object from the airway that you can see. *(Zucker, p. 380)*

21.

D. Your role is to prevent the patient from injuring himself or herself. *(Zucker, p. 341)*

22.

D. You should prevent the patient from injuring himself or herself. *(Zucker, p. 341)*

23.

B. An aura is a signal—a smell or sensation—that always occurs before the patient has a seizure. *(Zucker, p. 341)*

24.

C. A grand mal seizure involves significant bodily motion while the body is stiff and the patient is unconscious. *(Zucker, p. 341)*

25.

A. Petit mal seizures are much less dramatic physically than grand mal seizures and last usually less than 30 seconds. *(Zucker, p. 341)*

26.

C. Never try to move a patient who is having a seizure or force his or her mouth open to insert anything. Turning the patient's head for drainage will prevent aspiration. *(Zucker, p. 341)*

27.

D. Clean the patient of any saliva or vomitus. Never use restraints on a patient who is having a seizure. Avoid drink just after a seizure, until the patient is fully conscious and aware of activities. Notify your supervisor. *(Zucker, p. 341)*

28.

C. First be certain that the patient is actually choking or his or her airway is obstructed. *(Zucker, p. 378)*

29.

D. The objective is to expel the object. Each thrust should be separate and distinct. *(Zucker, p. 379)*

30.

B. The Heimlich maneuver is preferred after you determine that the patient has a complete airway obstruction. *(Zucker, pp. 378–379)*

31.

B. This is a good indication that the airway is completely obstructed. *(Zucker, p. 378)*

32.

B. Abdominal thrusts are a series of quick movements to the upper abdominal area. *(Zucker, p. 379)*

33.

D. In the Heimlich maneuver, the arms are placed around the person's waist, just in the middle of the upper abdomen. *(Zucker, p. 379)*

34.

A. The home care aide should be standing behind the person. *(Zucker, p. 379)*

35.

A. With partial airway obstruction, some air passes to and from the lungs, but the conditions must be improved. Snoring sounds may be noted. *(Zucker, p. 378)*

36.

C. Do not move the person unless she or he is in great danger of further injury. Do not leave the person who needs help. Oxygen is not readily available as common first aid. *(Zucker, p. 375–376)*

37.

B. If you have to perform artificial breathing, a pocket face shield will protect you. *(Zucker, p. 377)*

38.

A. If you do not see the object, do not sweep the mouth. If you see the foreign object, use your little finger in a hooking motion to remove it. *(Zucker, pp. 378–379)*

39.

C. Do not use back blows on a child. Abdominal thrusts are performed on a child similarly to the way they are used on adults. Call for assistance immediately. *(Zucker, p. 378)*

40.

B. Mouth-to-mouth ventilation (rescue breathing) should include 10 to 12 breaths per minute. *(Zucker, p. 381)*

41.

A. Infants and small children have higher oxygen demands than adults, and rescue breathing is one breath every 3 seconds. *(Zucker, p. 381)*

42.

C. Severe blood loss or excessive bleeding from a cut is called hemorrhage. *(Zucker, p. 382)*

43.

C. Capillaries feed the surface of the skin and will bleed when nicked by a razor. *(Zucker, pp. 103, 382)*

44.

B. Veins have low blood pressure. Any laceration to a vein would result in oozing blood. *(Zucker, pp. 103, 382)*

45.

A. Arteries are under high blood pressure. Any damage from the outside to an artery would result in profuse, spurting bleeding. *(Zucker, pp. 103, 382)*

46.

C. Tourniquets are not used as first aid to treat external blood loss. *(Zucker, p. 382)*

47.

B. Shock is the failure of the heart and vascular system to pump enough blood to all parts of the body, often as a result of severe blood loss. *(Zucker, pp. 384–385)*

48.

C. Expert medical help is essential. Stay with the patient. Do not give anything by mouth to the unconscious patient. *(Zucker, p. 383)*

49.

D. Chemicals and gases, when inhaled, may even cause difficulty seeing, hearing, and speaking; hallucinations; or collapse. *(Zucker, p. 383)*

50.

C. Insect bites can cause allergic reactions, and these are signs of allergic reaction. *(Zucker, p. 384)*

51.

A. The face is pale and may be bluish in color. *(Zucker, p. 384)*

52.

C. Facilitate blood flow to the brain as much as possible. Keep the person warm. *(Zucker, pp. 384–385)*

53.

B. Second degree burns cause blistering. *(Zucker, p. 385)*

54.

A. Burns may severely alter the person's body image and life. *(Zucker, p. 386)*

55.

B. Cool water will slow the progression of the burn and reduce the pain. *(Zucker, p. 386)*

56.

D. Do not wet the dressing. This will chill the person and cause shock. *(Zucker, p. 386)*

57.

C. Most heart attacks do not follow unusual physical activity but occur during sleep. *(Zucker, p. 386)*

58.

B. The pulse will be rapid and weak. *(Zucker, p. 387)*

59.

B. Do not give the heart attack victim anything to eat or drink. *(Zucker, p. 387)*

60.

A. The person may have paralysis in an extremity. *(Zucker, p. 387)*

12 Personal Hygiene and Grooming

chapter objectives

Upon completion of Chapter 12, the student is responsible for the following:

- ➤ Define oral hygiene.
- ➤ Define complete bed bath.
- ➤ Define partial bath.
- ➤ Define tub bath.
- ➤ Define shower.
- ➤ Define back rub.
- ➤ Define hair care, including shampoo.
- ➤ Define shaving.

DIRECTIONS
Each of the questions or incomplete statements below is followed by four suggested answers or completions. Select **one answer** that is best in each case.

1. When giving a bed bath, you position the patient on the side of the bed closest to you because it will:
   A. encourage communication
   B. allow you to use good body mechanics
   C. provide more security for the patient
   D. increase your ability to observe the patient

2. In what order do you wash the patient's extremities when giving a bed bath?
   A. Wash the extremity farthest from you first.
   B. Wash the extremity closest to you first.
   C. Wash the extremities last.
   D. Wash the extremities first.

3. Which of the following statements is/are true regarding the water in the bath basin?
   A. The basin should be one-fourth full.
   B. The water temperature should be checked with your whole hand.
   C. The water should be changed every 10 minutes.
   D. all of the above

4. In giving a bed bath, the time to offer the bedpan or urinal is:
   A. before staring the bed bath
   B. before washing the perineum
   C. at the end of the bed bath
   D. after washing the perineum

5. Privacy can be provided for the patient during the bed bath by:
   A. asking family or visitors to leave the room
   B. using a blanket to keep the patient covered
   C. removing the top sheet from underneath the blanket
   D. all of the above

6. If the patient starts complaining of pain during the bath, it is best to:
   A. give pain medication before continuing the bath
   B. make the water temperature warmer to increase relaxation
   C. stop the bath and make the patient comfortable
   D. all of the above

7. When washing the patient's face, it is best to:
   A. use lotion instead of soap
   B. use cold water instead of warm
   C. wash the eyes from the nose to the outside of the face
   D. all of the above

8. Which of the following is/are part of the procedure to wash an extremity?
   A. Place a towel lengthwise under the extremity.
   B. Support the joint of the extremity with the palm of your hand.
   C. Use long, firm strokes.
   D. all of the above

9. Which part of the body is washed last during a bed bath?
   A. the genital area
   B. the feet
   C. the back
   D. the axilla

10. A major concern in changing the linen on the bed is to:
    A. put on clean sheets every day
    B. take the sheets directly to the washer
    C. check for personal items before placing the sheets in the wash
    D. check for stains before placing the sheets in the wash

11. A partial bath is one in which:
    A. the patient can assist you with the bathing
    B. only a portion of the patient's body is washed
    C. the patient can take a shower with assistance
    D. the patient can take a tub bath with assistance

12. When assisting your patient to take any type of bath, the first thing you do is:
    A. check the mental status of your patient
    B. assemble your equipment
    C. remove all electric appliances from the bathroom
    D. fill the tub half full of water

13. Which of the following statements is true relating to bathing the patient?
    A. The type of bath given is the patient's choice.
    B. Establish a daily bathing routine.
    C. Specific instructions from the supervisor are needed for a tub bath or shower.
    D. Have the patient's family assist with the bathing.

14. Which safety factors should be remembered in assisting a patient with a tub bath or shower?
    A. Remove all electrical appliances from the bathroom.
    B. Check the grab bars in the bath or shower.
    C. Provide a nonskid bathmat.
    D. all of the above

15. Washing the patient's hair should be done:
    A. when giving the patient a tub bath
    B. daily with the shower
    C. when your supervisor gives you instructions
    D. at the sink

16. You inspect your patient's head before shampooing and find what you believe to be lice on your patient's head. You should:
    A. notify your supervisor immediately
    B. wear gloves and wash the patient's head with special shampoo for lice
    C. notify the patient's family so that they can check each other
    D. all of the above

17. Guidelines for hair care include:
    A. using only new packaged permanents
    B. styling the patient's hair with a curling iron the way she wants to wear it
    C. keeping the patient free of drafts when shampooing
    D. all of the above

18. The correct procedure for washing the patient's hair is to:
    A. apply shampoo, wet the hair, lather, then rinse
    B. wet the hair, apply shampoo, use both hands, and massage the scalp with the fingernails
    C. wet the hair, lather with shampoo, use both hands to wash, and massage the scalp with the fingertips
    D. wet the hair, apply shampoo, rinse, and apply conditioner

19. In shampooing a patient's hair in bed, it is best to:
    A. position the head over the side of the bed with the basin on the floor
    B. use a plastic bag and make a trough under the patient's head
    C. place rolled-up bath towels on each side and under the patient's head
    D. place a pillow under the patient's neck and rest the head in the basin

20. When shaving a patient, you should:
    A. use an electric razor if the patient is receiving oxygen
    B. use upward strokes over the cheeks
    C. put medication on the area if you nick the patient's skin
    D. none of the above

21. Wearing gloves when shaving a patient with a safety razor:
    A. is a standard precaution
    B. is not necessary, since there are no bodily fluids on the face
    C. is optional based on the patient's diagnosis
    D. cannot be done if you are to hold the skin taut

22. Which of the following are guidelines for shaving a patient with a safety razor?
    A. Position the patient with the head rest flat or in a lying position.
    B. Apply shaving cream generously to the face.
    C. Use long, firm, downward strokes to shave the neck under the chin.
    D. none of the above

23. The best time to inspect the patient's fingernails and toenails is:
    A. at the end of the day when swelling and other problems are more noticeable
    B. when assisting the patient to dress
    C. during bath time
    D. when trimming the nails

24. Your patient complains that his feet feel as if they are burning some of the time. They appear very red before you help him to the shower but look normal when you help him put his socks on. What should you do about his complaint?
    A. report to your supervisor immediately
    B. write the information down so that you can report it when checking out with your supervisor

C. ask his family to get a foot fungus medication
D. scrub the shower floor with a strong disinfectant

25. Your patient has a dark blue quarter-sized spot on the bottom of her big toe. The best plan of action for you is to:
    A. report to your supervisor immediately
    B. write it in your notes so that you can report it when checking out with your supervisor
    C. ask her family to get her new house shoes
    D. wash the area with mild soap and water

26. A back massage is routinely given with the bed bath to:
    A. stimulate circulation
    B. provide for relaxation for the patient
    C. prevent pressure sores
    D. all of the above

27. The primary cause of skin breakdown is:
    A. low pulse, which causes poor circulation
    B. letting patients who have had a stroke lie on their back
    C. pressure on bony prominences
    D. all of the above

28. Problems that are seen in the skin of elderly patients include:
    A. dry, rough skin
    B. loss of skin tone
    C. decrease in circulation to the skin
    D. all of the above

29. Observation of the skin includes:
    A. temperature
    B. cleanliness
    C. dryness
    D. all of the above

30. An open wound that occurs from decreased circulation due to pressure is called:

A. a decubitus ulcer

B. an ulcerated blister

C. a circulation sore

D. a pressure indentation

31. A good way to prevent shearing is to:
    A. place cornstarch on the sheets
    B. immobilize the joint
    C. use sheepskin or egg-crate padding
    D. all of the above

32. Bed sores can be caused by:
    A. shearing
    B. allowing the patient to stay in bed 24 hours a day
    C. allowing the patient to stay on one side for two hours
    D. all of the above

33. If not cared for properly, an area of the skin that is hot to the touch, red, and tender that does not go away will next change to:
    A. gray in color, then a blister, then an open wound
    B. an open wound with drainage
    C. an infected wound
    D. red, draining blister

34. A decubitus ulcer can be prevented by:
    A. keeping the patient clean and dry
    B. turning the patient every 2 hours
    C. keeping the bottom sheet free of wrinkles
    D. all of the above

35. If a patient is incontinent, the best way to protect the skin is to:
    A. use rubber pants to keep the urine and feces contained
    B. use bed protectors
    C. clean the patient immediately
    D. all of the above

36. Your 81-year-old patient had a stroke and is paralyzed on the left side. She is very thin, so measures to prevent decubiti from forming include:
    A. elbow pads
    B. heel egg-crate booties
    C. keeping her clean and dry
    D. all of the above

37. When caring for an incontinent patient, you should:
    A. ask the family to buy disposable products for him or her to wear
    B. use a generous amount of powder on the perineum
    C. wash the area to remove all urine and feces
    D. all of the above

38. Which of the following statements best describes skin care for a patient with a decubitus ulcer?
    A. The doctor will prescribe medication for the ulcer.
    B. Skin care will be based on the patient's size and physical condition.
    C. Skin care is a 24-hour concern.
    D. Egg-crate or sheepskin protectors must be used.

39. Your patient has dry, cracked skin on his feet, so it is important that you:
    A. use lotion on the affected areas
    B. wash the feet daily with mild soap and water
    C. report this to your supervisor
    D. use over-the-counter medication for the cracked areas

40. Skin problems on the feet may be caused by:
    A. poor hygiene
    B. chronic diseases such as diabetes
    C. decreased physical activity
    D. all of the above

41. Observations about the feet that should be reported to your supervisor include:
    A. tingling or other changes in sensation in the feet
    B. changes in color or temperature
    C. toenails that are curling into the toes
    D. all of the above

42. Your patient is having swelling of the feet and legs. You should:
    A. elevate the feet and legs and notify your supervisor
    B. cover the feet with socks and call your supervisor
    C. apply an ice pack and notify your supervisor
    D. all of the above

43. When caring for a patient receiving radiation therapy, you should:
    A. wash the area with cool water
    B. not use lotions on the red areas of the skin within the marked areas
    C. report changes in the skin within the marked areas
    D. all of the above

44. Which of the following should be reported immediately about your patient who is receiving radiation therapy?
    A. The skin within the marked lines is broken.
    B. The patient is shaving the marked area with an electric razor.
    C. The skin appears very red within the marked treatment lines.
    D. The marks on the skin for the treatment cannot be taken off with soap.

45. When giving care to a patient who is receiving chemotherapy, the area needing the most care is usually:
    A. the feet
    B. the mouth
    C. the hair
    D. the eyes

46. When caring for a patient with dentures, you should:
    A. brush the patient's gums with a soft toothbrush when dentures are removed for cleaning
    B. use a special denture toothbrush for cleaning the dentures
    C. soak the dentures in a special solution each day
    D. encourage the patient to keep the dentures out as long as possible

47. Oral hygiene is best described as:
    A. mouth care given to an unconscious patient
    B. brushing the patient's teeth after each meal
    C. cleaning of the mouth, gums, teeth, or dentures
    D. prevention of tooth decay and gum disease

48. When giving oral hygiene to an unconscious patient, it is best to:
    A. use only a small amount of water in rinsing the patient's mouth
    B. use a tongue blade to hold the mouth open while using a soft-bristled brush with toothpaste
    C. tell the patient what you are going to do
    D. all of the above

49. When you finish giving oral hygiene to an unconscious patient, you must:
    A. sweep the inside of the mouth with your fingers to be sure no food particles remain
    B. place a small amount of lubricant on the patient's lips
    C. wrap the dentures in a paper tissue
    D. all of the above

50. When you must wash the patient's dentures, it is very important that you:
    A. place a washcloth in the sink and hold the dentures over it to wash them
    B. grasp the dentures firmly between your thumb and little finger

C. dry the dentures thoroughly before replacing them in the patient's mouth

D. all of the above

51. When giving personal care, you should wear gloves:

A. any time you may be exposed to bodily fluids

B. as a standard precaution

C. when the patient's diagnosis is uncertain

D. when the patient's diagnosis is a condition that you could get

52. In assisting a patient to dress, an injured limb is:

A. held at a right angle to the joint

B. held straight and supported at the joint

C. put into the garment last and taken out first

D. put into the garment first and taken out last

53. When assisting the patient with toileting, you should document your observations, but you would call your supervisor to report:

A. mucus in the urine

B. pain or burning on urination

C. difficulty in starting to urinate

D. all of the above

54. It is important to ask your patients about their frequency and normal time to have a bowel movement because:

A. the number of stools a day varies from one patient to another

B. elimination of body waste is necessary to maintain a healthy body

C. this is a topic they might not begin to discuss with you

D. all of the above

55. In helping a patient with a bedpan, comfort can be increased by:

A. warming the bedpan

B. placing a pillow under the small of the patient's back

C. keeping the head of the bed flat

D. all of the above

56. If a patient is unable to lift his buttocks to get on or off the bedpan, you should:

A. ask a family member to help you place the bedpan

B. place the patient on the bedpan when your supervisor is there to assist

C. have the patient turn on his side, put the bedpan against the buttocks, and have him turn back onto the bedpan

D. place two bed protectors under the patient, and have him defecate on them.

57. If a specimen is not needed, what measures can you take before the patient uses the bedpan to make cleaning it easier?

A. place several sheets of toilet tissue in the bottom of the pan

B. put a small amount of a disinfectant solution in the bedpan

C. place a disposable glove in the bottom of the pan

D. warm the bedpan by rinsing with warm water first

58. If a patient is able to be out of bed but cannot walk to the bathroom, you could assist the patient to use:

A. a portable commode

B. the urinal while standing at the bedside

C. a bedpan placed on a chair at the bedside

D. all of the above

59. If a male patient is unable to put a urinal in place, you should:

A. hold the patient's hand around his penis and assist him to place it in the urinal

B. place the patient's penis into the opening of the urinal as far as it will go

C. slide the urinal under the penis and let it rest in the opening of the urinal

D. ask a male member of the family to assist him

60. After assisting the patient with using a urinal, you should chart:
    A. the color, amount, and any odor of the urine
    B. the time the patient voided
    C. the fact that a urinal was used
    D. all of the above

61. After assisting the patient with elimination, you should:
    A. have the patient wash his or her hands
    B. allow the patient to rest for a few minutes
    C. have the patient drink a full glass of water
    D. offer a warm liquid, such as coffee

62. When assisting a patient with a bedpan, you should put on gloves:
    A. after you have washed your hands
    B. when you take the bedpan to empty it
    C. when you place the bedpan under the patient
    D. when you wipe the patient

63. The purpose of using a peri bottle for perineal care is to:
    A. keep from having to touch the patient's perineum
    B. prevent contamination of the perineum
    C. apply medicated solution to the patient's perineum
    D. provide cleansing without damaging the skin

64. The perineum is the area:
    A. between the labia on the female
    B. from the pubic hair to the rectum
    C. between the anus and the external genital organs
    D. between the urinary meatus and the anus

65. When drying the perineum, you should gently wipe:
    A. from front to back
    B. from back to front
    C. from side to side
    D. from the cleanest area to the dirtiest

66. The best solution to use in cleansing the perineum is:
    A. mild soap and water
    B. diluted astringent
    C. a medicated solution
    D. warm water

67. Perineal care is given:
    A. following childbirth
    B. after perineal surgery
    C. for cleansing when a bath or shower are not taken
    D. all of the above

68. Which of the following apply to performing all procedures on a patient?
    A. Wash your hands and put on gloves.
    B. Ask family members or visitors to leave the room.
    C. Explain the procedure to the patient.
    D. all of the above

69. Your patient is having frequent, small, black, sticky bowel movements. You should:
    A. notify your supervisor
    B. encourage more fluids by mouth
    C. change your patient's diet
    D. restrict the amount of red meat that is eaten

70. Negligence is a legal term. In which of the following situations would the home care aide be guilty of negligence?
    A. writing down the wrong time you gave the patient a tub bath
    B. refusing to give the patient a permanent for her hair
    C. not providing for the patient's scheduled personal hygiene
    D. all of the above

71. The patient has a daily shower ordered but says that her skin is too dry and wants to shower only twice a week. You should:

A. explain the importance of a daily shower and get her some skin lotion

B. allow the patient to shower twice a week and wash the genital area and under the arms daily

C. explain that you are held responsible for giving her a shower every day

D. call your supervisor and report that the patient is not cooperative

72. When giving your patient a tub bath, the patient slips and bumps his knee on the edge of the tub. You should:

A. chart it and call your supervisor

B. put ice on the knee to keep it from swelling and chart it

C. call your supervisor and complete an incident report

D. call the doctor so that the patient's knee can be X-rayed

73. When bathing your new patient, you discover bruises on both arms and one on his thigh. You should:

A. not use soap over the bruised areas

B. chart your observations and call your supervisor

C. ask the family how the patient got the bruises

D. all of the above

74. When providing mouth care for the unconscious patient, the home care aide should:

A. rinse her mouth with lots of mouthwash

B. force her mouth open if needed

C. choose a toothbrush with soft bristles and rinse with lots of water

D. position the patient's head to the side to prevent aspiration

75. In bathing the patient, the water should be:

A. hot

B. warm

C. cool

D. however the patient likes it

76. If a patient cannot perform his or her own oral hygiene, the home care aide should help the patient to do this:

A. once a day

B. twice a day

C. after sweets, such as candy

D. twice a day and after every meal prn

77. Which of the following statements about perineal care is true?

A. You should always do perineal care for your patients.

B. Perineal care is not required for males.

C. It is important to encourage a patient to do his or her own perineal care.

D. Perineal care is done only when a patient is incontinent.

78. When you help a patient with bathing and shampooing in a bathtub, check the water temperature with:

A. your whole hand

B. your elbow

C. the patient's hand

D. the patient's elbow

79. When shaving a patient, the home care aide should:

A. wash hands and wear disposable gloves

B. use a disinfectant on the patient's face before shaving him

C. shave opposite to the direction of hair growth

D. rinse the razor as little as possible to avoid dulling the blade

80. Dentures should be brushed thoroughly at least:

A. every 2 hours

B. every 4 hours

C. every 12 hours

D. every 24 hours

81. When the patient is using a shower, the home care aide should:
    A. stay with the patient
    B. check on the patient every 5 minutes
    C. have the patient call when finished
    D. leave the patient alone to bathe in privacy

82. An important consideration in bathing the patient is to:
    A. encourage assistance by family members
    B. observe safety rules
    C. use as little water as possible to avoid waste
    D. all of the above

83. When cleaning the patient's dentures, you should:
    A. line the sink with a washcloth or paper towel
    B. use an abrasive cleanser to remove all debris
    C. soak the dentures 12 hours each day
    D. all of the above

84. When providing oral hygiene to the unconscious patient, you should do all of the following except:
    A. position the patient on his side
    B. put your fingers in his or her mouth
    C. rinse with small amounts of water
    D. apply lubricant to his lips

85. Your patient, Miss Mabry, is to have a complete bed bath during your visit today. You should begin washing with:
    A. her arms
    B. her face
    C. her feet
    D. her back

86. The patient's hair can be shampooed in bed in all of the following situations except when:
    A. the patient is bedbound
    B. the patient has a fever
    C. the patient has recently had a stroke
    D. the patient has just had hip surgery

87. When providing nail care for a patient, the home care aide may do all of the following except:
    A. cut the nails
    B. soak the nails
    C. clean with an orange stick
    D. file the nails straight across

88. The purpose of the bed bath is to:
    A. remove waste products from the skin
    B. warm the patient
    C. minimize skin circulation
    D. All of the above

89. You are providing oral hygiene to your patient. All of the following observations should be reported except:
    A. lip cracks
    B. odor
    C. decubitus
    D. gum sores

90. All of the following observations after hair care should be reported except:
    A. sores
    B. lice
    C. healthy hair
    D. excessive dandruff

91. While assisting a patient with a tub bath, the home care aide should do all of the following except:
    A. fill the bathtub half full with water
    B. leave the patient alone
    C. check grab bars
    D. remove all electric appliances from the bathroom

92. All of the following equipment is necessary to give a bed bath except:
    A. bath mat
    B. bath blanket
    C. wash basin
    D. towels

93. Mr. Denton has a broken right collarbone. When assisting him with dressing, the home care aide should:
    A. select his clothing for the day
    B. assist him to dress his right arm first
    C. leave him alone to dress
    D. drape his shirt across his back

94. Once you have finished cleaning the patient's dentures, you should store them:
    A. wrapped in tissue
    B. on the bedside table
    C. in a marked denture cup
    D. in the medicine cabinet

95. Dentures should be cleaned with:
    A. antiseptic mouthwash
    B. toothpaste or denture cleanser
    C. soap and hot water
    D. cold water and dental floss

96. You are to assist your patient with a shower. You must protect the patient from:
    A. infection
    B. aspiration
    C. falling
    D. fainting

97. You are giving Mrs. Eaton a bed bath and note a red spot on her right heel. You should:

A. rub the area vigorously with lotion
B. report your observation to her daughter
C. report your observation to the supervisor
D. place sheepskin under her heels

98. The best way to use a washcloth during a bed bath is to:
    A. form a mitten
    B. fold it into fourths
    C. roll it up into a ball
    D. hold it loosely

99. Mrs. Faulkner asks to have her hair shampooed. The home care aide should:
    A. tell the family to call a beautician
    B. suggest that brushing and combing be done instead
    C. report this request to your nurse supervisor
    D. get the equipment and prepare to give a shampoo in bed

100. As you prepare to shampoo your patient's hair in bed, you should assemble all of the following equipment except:
    A. the patient's shampoo
    B. a pitcher
    C. a water trough
    D. a spray nozzle

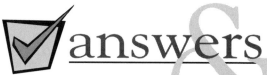

answers & rationales

1.

B. Keeping your work close to your body is a principle of good body mechanics. *(Zucker, p. 210)*

2.

A. Starting with the extremity farthest from you is the recommended procedure. *(Zucker, p. 211)*

3.

B. The whole hand is more sensitive to water temperature than the fingers. The basin should be two-thirds full and the water changed as necessary to maintain the temperature and keep it clean. *(Zucker, p. 211)*

4.

A. The patient will be more comfortable during the bath if the bedpan is offered first. *(Zucker, p. 210)*

5.

D. Privacy includes no visitiors during the bath, keeping the body covered except for the part being washed, and not exposing the patient while you remove the top sheet. *(Zucker, p. 210)*

6.

C. Any time a patient becomes tired or uncomfortable, stop the bath. Changing water temperature will not help to relieve pain, and the home health aide should not give pain medication to the patient. *(Zucker, p. 210)*

7.

C. The eyes are washed as described; warm water is used to wash the face, with soap if the patient wishes. *(Zucker, p. 211)*

8.

D. The towel keeps the bed from getting wet, the support of the joint prevents strain, and the long, firm strokes are appropriate. *(Zucker, p. 210)*

9.

A. The genitalia are always washed last. The feet are washed as each leg is washed, and the water is changed before washing the back, which is the next-to-last area to be washed. *(Zucker, p. 212)*

10.

C. Personal items can easily be bundled into sheets, so check for things like glasses, dentures, watches, and jewelry before you put sheets in the washer. *(Zucker, p. 203)*

11.

A. A partial bath refers to the patient taking an active part in bathing as much of the body as can safely be reached or as much as can be tolerated alone. Shower and tub baths are not called partial baths. *(Zucker, p. 212)*

12.

B. For your patient's safety and comfort, you assemble the equipment needed first. Other options are used only for giving the patient a tub bath or shower. *(Zucker, pp. 210–213)*

13.

C. A bed bath or partial bath is given unless your supervisor approves a tub bath or shower. Answer A is not appropriate, since the type of bath may depend on the patient's diagnosis. Not every patient needs a bath each day and the patient's privacy may be invaded if family members helped. *(Zucker, p. 213)*

14.

D. Electrical appliances must be removed to remove the possibility of electrical shock; grab bars could be loose; the nonskid bathmat is needed for the tub and shower. *(Zucker, pp. 214–215)*

15.

C. A specific order is needed before you shampoo the patient's hair, and the supervisor will say when and where to do it. *(Zucker, p. 216)*

16.

A. Calling the supervisor should be done immediately so that you will know how to proceed. It is not within your role to get the lice shampoo without specific instructions or to notify the family. *(Zucker, p. 217)*

17.

C. You must protect the patient from drafts while the head is wet because most of body heat is lost through the head. Never give a patient a permanent or use a curling iron on the patient's hair. *(Zucker, p. 217)*

18.

C. The hair should be wet before applying the shampoo, both hands are used to wash the hair and massage the scalp, but fingertips are used, never fingernails. A conditioner may or may not be used. *(Zucker, p. 218)*

19.

B. The plastic bag trough will allow the water to drain away from the head and keep the patient driest. The position of the patient in the other options would not be comfortable and would not maintain good body alignment. *(Zucker, p. 217)*

20.

D. Never use an electric razor if oxygen is going, as it may cause a spark and start a fire; use downward strokes over the face; do not put any medication on the patient. *(Zucker, p. 221)*

21.

A. Wear gloves when giving personal care as a standard precaution. The possiblility of contact with blood and body fluids exists if the patient is nicked by the safety razor. *(Zucker, p. 221)*

22.

B. A lot of shaving cream reduces friction and decreases the chance of irritating the patient's face. The patient's head should be up if possible; use short, firm, upward strokes under the chin. *(Zucker, p. 221)*

23.

C. It is easiest to inspect the nails when bathing the patient. The time of day is not as important, and you should not cut the patient's nails. *(Zucker, p. 211)*

24.

B. Document and report any changes in sensation on skin or feet; since this is not an emergency, it can be reported at the end of the day. Neither foot medication nor scrubbing with a disinfectant may be neccessary. *(Zucker, p. 199)*

25.

A. Changes in color to dark blue or red may indicate a lack of circulation and should be reported immediately. New house shoes or washing the area will not improve circulation. *(Zucker, p. 199)*

26.

D. Backrubs provide all of these benefits. *(Zucker, p. 215)*

27.

C. Skin breakdown is caused by pressure on body parts, especially bony prominences; they can occur regardless of pulse rate or patient diagnosis. *(Zucker, p. 192)*

28.

D. As skin ages, all of these changes occur. *(Zucker, p. 193)*

29.

D. All of these observations should be included each time you visit a patient. *(Zucker, p. 193)*

30.

A. Decubitus ulcers, also called bedsores or pressure sores, occur where skin is broken because of pressure. *(Zucker, p. 197)*

31.

A. Cornstarch placed directly on sheets decreases friction and allows the patient to move without shearing. Sheepskins, egg-crates, and joint immobilizers will not prevent shearing. *(Zucker, p. 193)*

32.

A. Shearing can cause skin breakdown that leads to decubitus ulcers. Patients on bedrest must remain in bed 24 hours a day and should be turned every 2 hours. *(Zucker, p. 193)*

33.

A. Progression in decubitus ulcers is from red to gray to blister formation, then to an open wound. Infections or drainage may occur later. *(Zucker, p. 197)*

34.

D. All of these are effective methods for preventing decubitus ulcer formation. *(Zucker, pp. 195–196)*

35.

C. Incontinent patients should be kept clean and dry, no matter how often you must clean them and change the bed. Rubber pants are irritating to the skin. Bed protectors keep the linens protected but do not protect the patient's skin. *(Zucker, p. 195)*

36.

D. All of these measures can be used to protect bony prominences from pressure. *(Zucker, p. 193)*

37.

C. Keep incontinent patients clean and dry; use powder sparingly because it cakes in body creases. Discuss disposable products with your supervisor before recommending that they be purchased. *(Zucker, p. 195)*

38.

C. Skin care must occur all day every day and must be shared by all caregivers. The other options may or may not be true of patients with decubitus ulcers. *(Zucker, p. 198)*

39.

C. Observe and report changes in feet to your supervisor. The patient may not notice these changes. Do not apply any treatment to areas without your supervisor's instructions. *(Zucker, p. 199)*

40.

D. All of these situations can contribute to skin problems on a patient's feet. *(Zucker, p. 199)*

41.

D. All of these things should be observed and reported to your supervisor. *(Zucker, p. 199)*

42.

A. The immediate action to take for swollen feet and legs is to elevate them on a chair or couch; then report the situation to your supervisor. Swelling of feet and legs can indicate a worsening heart condition. *(Zucker, p. 200)*

43.

D. All of these actions are appropriate care for a patient receiving radiation therapy. The skin in the area marked for radiation is very fragile and should be washed gently with cool water. Observe for skin changes, and avoid using lotion on the skin in the marked area. *(Zucker, p. 200)*

44.

A. Skin within these marks is being teated with radiation. A break in the skin is serious. The marks should be left in place and, in fact, cannot be washed off. It is considered normal if the area within the marks becomes red. The area can be shaved with an electric razor if needed. *(Zucker, p. 200)*

45.

B. Chemotherapy can cause a sore, dry mouth and throat, which must be cleansed gently. The eyes and feet are not affected, although the patient's hair may fall out. *(Zucker, p. 201)*

46.

A. Gums should be stimulated with a soft toothbrush when dentures are removed. Dentures can be cleaned by using an ordinary toothbrush and are generally soaked at night. Dentures should be worn as desired by the patient. *(Zucker, p. 205)*

47.

C. Oral hygiene involves keeping the mouth, gums, teeth, and dentures clean. This is done for conscious and unconscious patients to prevent disease. *(Zucker, p. 204)*

48.

C. Even if the patient is unconscious, he or she still may hear you. Toothpaste and water should never be used for an unconscious patient because of the danger of choking. *(Zucker, p. 207)*

49.

B. Lubricant will keep the unconscious patient's lips moist. To avoid the chance of being bitten, do not place your fingers inside the patient's mouth. *(Zucker, p. 207)*

50.

A. Lining the sink with a paper towel or washcloth will cushion dentures if they fall. Hold dentures securely, and rinse them before replacing them in the patient's mouth. *(Zucker, p. 206)*

51.

B. Standard precautions state that gloves must be worn when contact is possible with blood, all body fluids except sweat, broken skin, and all mucous membranes. This includes activities during direct care. *(Zucker, p. 124)*

52.

D. An injured or rigid extremity is first into a garment and last out. None of the other choices will be effective in dressing a patient with an injured limb. *(Zucker, p. 208)*

53.

D. All of these observations indicate a problem and should be reported and documented. *(Zucker, p. 222)*

54.

D. All of these are reasons you need to ask about bowel movements rather than expect a patient to offer information on his or her own. *(Zucker, p. 222)*

55.

A. The bedpan should be warmed with warm water and placed beneath the buttocks, and the head of the bed should be elevated to a sitting position. *(Zucker, p. 223)*

56.

C. You can assist your patient onto the bedpan in this way without the assistance of another person. You should place the patient on a bedpan for defecation. *(Zucker, p. 223)*

57.

A. Placing sheets of toilet tissue or a slight bit of water in the bedpan will make it easier to clean. None of the other options is appropriate for making cleaning easier. *(Zucker, p. 223)*

58.

D. All of these are ways the patient can toilet without walking to the bathroom. *(Zucker, p. 222)*

59.

B. If the patient is unable to help himself, you must place his penis into the urinal and hold it in place while he urinates. Otherwise, urine may get on the patient, bed, and linens. *(Zucker, p. 224)*

60.

D. All of this information should be documented in the patient's chart. *(Zucker, p. 225)*

61.

A. The patient should always be given the opportunity to clean his or her hands after toileting for infection control purposes. The other options are not necessary for every patient. *(Zucker, pp. 224–226)*

62.

A. Put on gloves after you wash your hands and before obtaining the clean bedpan as part of standard precautions. *(Zucker, p. 223)*

63.

D. The perineal skin may be fragile after childbirth or surgery, and a washcloth could be too harsh to use in the area. A peribottle is used instead. *(Zucker, p. 226)*

64.

C. The perineal area on both males and females refers to the area between the anus and external genital organs. *(Zucker, p. 226)*

65.

A. Wiping from front to back prevents bacteria from the anal area from being wiped toward the vagina and urinary meatus, where it could cause infection. *(Zucker, p. 227)*

66.

A. Warm soapy water is placed in one peribottle, and warm clean water in the other bottle. The soapy water is used first, then the clean water. Medications and astringents should not be used on the perineal area unless ordered by a physician. *(Zucker, p. 227)*

67.

D. Pericare is given in all of these situations to promote cleansing and healing of the perineal area. *(Zucker, p. 226)*

68.

D. All of the steps are performed with every procedure. *(Zucker, pp. 204–227)*

69.

A. Report unusual color and frequency of patient's elimination to your supervisor. These symptoms may indicate a serious problem and should not be ignored. *(Zucker, p. 222)*

70.

C. Negligence means failure to give proper care when you know how to do so, which results in physical or emotional harm to the patient. Failure to provide scheduled personal hygiene is an example of negligence. *(Zucker, p. 13)*

71.

B. Patients do not need to have a complete bath or shower each day. Frequency depends on skin condition, climate, and patient preferences. *(Zucker, p. 209)*

72.

C. An accident or unusual happening is considered an incident. A report must be made and reported to the supervisor. This is done for the protection of the patient, yourself, and the agency. *(Zucker, p. 13)*

73.

B. Bruises can indicate many things. Try to determine when the bruise appeared, how big it is, and how long it lasts. It is not necessary to avoid using soap over the bruised areas, nor to question the family about how the bruises occurred. *(Zucker, p. 193)*

74.

D. Turning the patient's head to the side prevents aspiration of any liquids into the patient's lungs. *(Zucker, p. 207)*

75.

D. Ask the patient how he or she likes the water. Then, test it with your whole hand and let the patient test it with the inside of his or her hand. *(Zucker, p. 211)*

76.

D. This procedure should be done twice a day and after meals whenever possible. *(Zucker, p . 204)*

77.

C. This activity is usually done in private, so if the patient can perform his or her own perineal care, you should encourage him or her to do so. *(Zucker, p. 222)*

78.

A. First test with your whole hand, then permit the patient to check the temperature (to prevent the possibility of burning the patient). *(Zucker, p. 211)*

79.

A. Practice standard precautions if the risk of exposure to body fluids is possible, as in the case of shaving in which you may be exposed to blood if you accidentally nick the patient's skin. *(Zucker, p. 221)*

80.

C. Dentures should be brushed thoroughly at least once every 12 hours. *(Zucker, p. 205)*

81.

A. Safety is a key point with all patient care procedures, yet you should provide as much privacy as possible without leaving the patient alone. *(Zucker, p. 214)*

82.

B. Always observe safety rules with providing direct patient care. *(Zucker, p. 210)*

83.

A. Line the sink with a paper towel or washcloth so that if the dentures slip out of your hand, they will be cushioned as they fall. *(Zucker, p. 206)*

84.

B. Do not put your fingers in the patient's mouth. He or she may close the mouth and injure you. *(Zucker, p. 206)*

85.

B. The procedure for complete bed bath begins with washing the face first. *(Zucker, p. 211)*

86.

B. A fever indicates a sign of infection, and shampooing the hair in bed may cause the patient to be chilled and be quite uncomfortable. *(Zucker, p. 217)*

87.

A. Home care aides should never cut the patient's nails. If the skin is accidentally cut, many patients are at high risk for infection or additional injury. *(Zucker, p. 211)*

88.

A. Bathing takes waste products off the skin, along with many other beneficial effects. *(Zucker, p. 209)*

89.

C. The mouth is observed for cracks, sores, and odor. Decubitus ulcers appear on pressure points. *(Zucker, p. 204)*

90.

C. Healthy hair is not an abnormal observation. *(Zucker, p. 217)*

91.

B. Privacy is important, but the patient should be supervised closely to prevent accidents. *(Zucker, pp. 213–214)*

92.

A. A bath mat is used when you assist a patient with a tub bath or shower. *(Zucker, p. 210)*

93.

B. An injured arm (or leg) is first into a garment and last out. *(Zucker, p. 208)*

94.

C. Dentures are expensive; always put them in a carefully marked denture cup. *(Zucker, p. 205)*

95.

B. Dentures are to be cleaned with appropriate denture cleansers only. *(Zucker, p. 206)*

96.

C. Showers and bathrooms can be very slippery. Safety is always a top priority. *(Zucker, p. 211)*

97.

C. Report any abnormal observations to your supervisor, who can initiate actions to correct the problem(s). *(Zucker, p. 209)*

98.

A. Make a mitten with the washcloth throughout the bath procedure. *(Zucker, p. 211)*

99.

C. Be sure your supervisor has given you specific instructions to wash the patient's hair. *(Zucker, p. 216)*

100.

D. A hand-held spray nozzle would be used in a shower procedure. *(Zucker, p. 217)*

13 Transfers and Ambulation

chapter objectives

Upon completion of Chapter 13, the student is responsible for the following:

➤ Define guarding belt.

➤ Identify how to help a patient to sit up.

➤ Identify how to use a portable mechanical lift.

➤ Identify how to help a patient to stand.

➤ Identify how to perform a pivot transfer from bed to chair.

➤ Identify how to transfer from chair to bed.

➤ Describe ambulation activities.

➤ Describe assistive walking devices.

DIRECTIONS
Each of the questions or incomplete statements below is followed by four suggested answers or completions. Select **one answer** that is best in each case.

1. When assisting the patient from the bed to a chair, the chair should be placed:
   A. at a 45 degree angle to the bed so that the patient will move toward his or her stronger side
   B. at a 45 degree angle to the bed so that the patient will move toward his or her weaker side
   C. at a 90 degree angle to the bed so that the patient will move toward his or her stronger side
   D. at a 90 degree angle to the bed so that the patient will move toward his or her weaker side

2. To assist the patient from the bed to the chair, when the patient comes to a standing position, you should:
   A. place your foot near his or her foot for extra support
   B. keep your feet together for good body mechanics
   C. keep your feet between the patient's feet
   D. all of the above

3. Before helping a patient from the bed to a standing position, you should:
   A. place the patient's hand on the arm of the chair
   B. bring the patient to a sitting position with his or her legs over the side of the bed
   C. put the foot rests of the wheelchair in the up position
   D. all of the above

4. The term "ambulation" refers to:
   A. movement of the patient with assistance
   B. independent movement of the patient
   C. the action of walking
   D. assisting the patient with a special gait for walking

5. When the patient needs minimal assistance in ambulating, you should:
   A. stand on the strong side of the patient so that he or she can hold onto you
   B. stand on the weak side of the patient and support him or her with a guarding belt
   C. stand with one hand on the guarding belt and the other under the patient's axilla
   D. stand slightly in front of the patient with one hand on the guarding belt

6. When transferring a patient from the wheelchair to the bed, you should first:
   A. put the guarding belt on the patient
   B. pull up the foot rests on the wheelchair
   C. remove the patient's shoes
   D. lock the wheels on the chair

7. When assisting a patient to ambulate, you should stand:
   A. on the patient's weaker side and a little behind him or her
   B. with one hand on the guarding belt and your other hand in front of the collarbone on the weaker side
   C. with your feet about 12 inches apart for a firm base of support
   D. all of the above

8. When a patient needs minimal assistance in standing up from sitting in a chair, you should instruct the patient to:
   A. place his or her hands around your neck, place one foot in front of the other, and pull up on the count of three
   B. move to the front of the chair, place his or her hands on the arms of the chair, put one foot in under himself or herself, push down with his or her arms, lean forward, and stand up on the count of three
   C. hold onto your hands and, on the count of three, to pull up to a standing position
   D. place his or her arms around your waist when you put your knee between the

patient's legs and to stand when you rock back on your back foot on the count of three

9. When assisting a patient from the chair back to bed, the chair should be placed:

A. at a 45 degree angle to the bed so that the patient will move toward his or her stronger side

B. at a 45 degree angle to the bed so that the patient will move toward his or her weaker side

C. at a 90 degree angle to the bed so that the patient will move toward his or her stronger side

D. at a 90 degree angle to the bed so that the patient will move toward his or her weaker side

10. When reminding a patient how to walk up stairs on crutches, you will instruct the patient to:

A. advance the strongest leg to the next step, bring the weaker leg to the step, then the crutches

B. advance the weaker leg to the next step, bring the stronger leg to the step, then the crutches

C. advance the strongest leg to the next step, bring the crutches to the step and then the weaker leg.

D. advance the weaker leg to the next step, bring the crutches to the step and then the stronger leg

11. When walking down the stairs with a cane, the patient should:

A. advance the cane to the lower step, followed by the weaker leg and then the stronger one

B. advance the cane to the lower step, followed by the stronger leg and then the weaker one

C. advance the stronger leg to the lower step, followed by the cane and then the weaker leg.

D. advance the weaker leg to the lower step, followed by the stronger leg and then the cane

12. Which of the following statements is *not* true about using assistive walking devices?

A. Rubber tips should be on the ends of the canes, crutches, or walkers.

B. The hand piece of each assistive device should be level with the hip.

C. Use the walker or cane to pull up to a standing position.

D. There should be a slight bend at the elbow when the patient is standing with a cane or walker.

13. A cane is usually used on which side of the patient's body?

A. the weaker side

B. the side with the hand that the patient uses to write

C. the stronger side

D. the side opposite the hand that the patient uses to write

14. When walking with a cane, the patient will:

A. place the cane about 12 inches in front on his or her stronger side

B. bring the weaker leg forward so that it is even with the cane

C. bring the stronger leg forward just ahead of the cane

D. all of the above

15. When walking the standard three-point gait with crutches, the patient will:

A. place the crutches 8 to 12 inches in front of body with the weaker leg and bring the strong leg forward in front of crutches

B. bring the right foot and left crutch 8 to 12 inches forward, then bring the left foot and right crutch 8 to 12 inches forward

C. place the crutches 8 to 12 inches in front of body with the stronger leg and bring the weaker leg forward in front of crutches

D. bring the right crutch 8 to 12 inches forward, bring the left foot in front of crutch, bring left crutch in front of left foot, and bring the right foot in front of left foot

16. When assisting a patient to ambulate who is learning to use a crutch, you should:
    A. stand on the patient's weaker side and a little behind him or her
    B. stand on the patient's stronger side and a little behind him or her
    C. stand beside the patient on the stronger side
    D. stand slightly in front of the patient on his or her weaker side

17. The role of the homemaker or home health aide in caring for a patient who must learn to use an assistive walking device is to:
    A. teach the proper placement of the device and the gait to be used
    B. allow the physical therapist, registered nurse, or physician to be responsible for the patient's ability to properly and safely use the devices
    C. see that the patient uses the device properly and safely
    D. all of the above

18. Which of the following statements is/are true about the use of a walker?
    A. The patient should slide the walker along the ground, not pick up all four legs of the walker.
    B. If the walker is being moved, the patient's feet should be stationary.
    C. The right foot should be advanced with the walker, followed by the left foot.
    D. all of the above

19. Which of the following steps is not correct in helping the patient go from a standing position to a sitting position using assistive devices?
    A. Check to see that the chair is secured.
    B. Have the patient walk as close to the chair as possible and then turn his or her back to it with his or her legs against the chair.
    C. Have the patient hold the assistive device and lower himself or herself into the chair.
    D. none of the above

20. Which of the following observations should be charted about a patient who has been assisted from the bed to the chair and then back to bed?
    A. the time the patient stayed up in the chair
    B. any dizziness or other complaints
    C. the amount of assistance the patient needed
    D. all of the above

21. In assisting a patient to stand up, it is important to use the same sequence of actions each time because:
    A. the patient will be able to help to the level of his or her ability
    B. you can concentrate on helping the patient and not have to stop and remember whether you have said everything that was necessary
    C. a routine provides more security for the patient
    D. all of the above

22. The home should be inspected for environmental barriers that may prevent the patient from using assistive devices safely. These may include:
    A. chairs without arm rests
    B. narrow doorways
    C. furniture that does not allow for passage
    D. all of the above

23. When helping a patient to sit up on the bed, it is important for you to:
    A. use a wide base of support and keep your center of gravity close to the bed
    B. bend at your waist to roll the patient on to his or her side
    C. keep your weight on your front leg
    D. all of the above

24. In assisting a patient to ambulate, a guarding belt is useful for:
    A. helping you to pull the patient from a sitting to a standing position
    B. helping you to control the weaker side of the patient's body

C. giving you better control over the patient's center of gravity

D. all of the above

25. Which of the following types of chair provides the greatest amount of support for a patient who needs some assistance in moving?

A. a recliner

B. a large soft-cushioned chair

C. a dining room chair with arm rests

D. a chair that allows the feet to hang freely

26. When using a portable mechanical patient lift to get a patient from bed to a chair, you should:

A. turn the patient from side to side on the bed to place the sling under him or her

B. attach the sling to the mechanical lift with the hooks in place through the metal frame facing outward

C. align the back of the chair with the headboard of the bed

D. all of the above

27. When getting the patient up in a chair, the sling for the mechanical lift should be:

A. slid under the patient with the two hooks on the patient's right side removed

B. folded in half then rolled under the patient

C. left in the chair under the patient

D. all of the above

28. When the patient is in the sling being moved, you should:

A. guide the patient's legs

B. place a pillow under the patient's head

C. stay clear of the frame of the lift

D. all of the above

29. When you are unsure of how to help a patient who needs to be moved with the portable lift, it is best to:

A. wait for your supervisor to get the patient up

B. check with a reliable member of the family for the correct procedure

C. call your supervisor

D. not get the patient up until you have gone to a refresher inservice class

30. A patient refuses to use his cane for walking and tells you that he can do fine without it. What should you do?

A. Refuse to let the patient out of the chair without his cane.

B. Tell the family that you cannot be responsible for the patient if he does not use the cane.

C. Call your supervisor.

D. Allow the patient to do as he pleases.

31. Your patient appears somewhat confused when it is time to get out of bed and walk with a walker. You should:

A. keep the patient in bed

B. check the chart to see whether the patient has been confused before

C. call your supervisor

D. all of the above

32. The patient's family does not want you to get her out of bed now that she is napping because she did not sleep well last night. You should:

A. allow the patient to rest and get her up later

B. insist on getting the patient up so that she will sleep this night

C. explain the importance of getting the patient up to maintain muscle strength

D. call your supervisor

33. Negligence is a legal term. In which of the following situations would the home care aide be guilty of negligence?

A. if a patient fell to his knees when walking to the dining room table

B. if a patient did not ambulate as ordered for three days because she told you that she was too tired

C. if you did not allow a patient to use his crutches until the reported missing screws were replaced

D. all of the above

34. The patient's friend from the Senior Citizens' Center came to visit on crutches. The patient and his family agreed that the way the friend was using his crutches seemed more stable and easier than the way the physical therapist had instructed the patient. You should:
    A. tell the family to report this to their case manager
    B. tell the family that you will call the physical therapist
    C. explain that different gaits depend on the type of problem the person has but you will report their desires to your supervisor
    D. show the patient how to walk using the different gait, document it, and report it to the physical therapist

35. The family tells you that their friend's mother got a mechanical lift to get her out of bed. They want to know how to get one for their mother. You should:
    A. tell them that you will find out where they can order one
    B. tell them that you will check with their insurance to see whether a lift would be covered
    C. call and tell your supervisor of the situation
    D. all of the above

36. When assisting a patient from a chair back into bed, the patient should stand, reach for the bed, and pivot with your guidance. To pivot means to:
    A. turn
    B. bend
    C. stretch
    D. step up

37. The use of a guarding (transfer) belt is appropriate when:
    A. pulling the patient up in bed
    B. ambulating the patient
    C. turning the patient in bed
    D. all of the above

38. When transferring a patient from a bed to a wheelchair:
    A. unlock the brakes of the wheelchair
    B. keep the bed flat
    C. position the wheelchair close to the foot of the bed
    D. place the wheelchair so that the patient will move toward the stronger side

39. Which of the following is not an important question for the home care aide to ask herself or himself before moving a patient?
    A. Do I need help?
    B. Do I have all the equipment I need?
    C. Is the television turned off?
    D. Have I positioned myself so that I will not injure myself?

40. How should the home care aide apply a guarding (transfer) belt on the patient?
    A. Put it over the patient's clothing, around his or her midsection.
    B. Place it around the patient's chest.
    C. Put it on very tightly.
    D. Hold it closed with safety pins.

41. When assisting a patient with a weak left side from a wheelchair, the home care aide should give support to the:
    A. weak side
    B. strong side
    C. front side
    D. back side

42. When a patient is sitting in a chair, his or her back should:
    A. not touch the back of the chair
    B. be curved forward
    C. be supported by the back of the chair
    D. twist to one side

43. Which of the following is *not* an assistive device used for ambulation?
    A. walker
    B. gait belt

C. cane

D. mechanical lift

44. In assisting a patient to ambulate using a cane:

A. the cane should be moved 2 to 4 inches ahead of the patient

B. the patient should hold the cane on the weak side of the body

C. the patient should use the cane to stand

D. the patient should hold the cane on the strong side of the body

45. When transferring a patient from the bed to a chair, which of the following is appropriate technique?

A. lifting the patient to the chair

B. holding the patient around the chest

C. using a guarding (transfer) belt

D. using a walker to assist with the transfer

46. How often should the home care aide wash his or her hands during the transfer procedure?

A. before the procedure

B. after the procedure

C. hand washing is not necessary

D. before and after the procedure

47. Which of the following observations should be reported immediately after placing a patient in a wheelchair?

A. sudden weakness

B. coughing

C. sneezing

D. warm skin

48. A primary function of the physical therapist is to:

A. assist the patient with activities of motion

B. assist the patient with nutrition

C. assist the patient with performing ADLs

D. assist the patient with aphasia

49. A walker is used:

A. when one or both legs need to regain strength

B. to support a weak body part

C. to provide support when there is a weakness on one side of the body

D. to provide a safer and more secure support than a cane

50. You are assisting your patient with ambulation. You should:

A. stand on the patient's weaker side and a little behind him or her

B. encourage the patient to walk rapidly

C. encourage the patient to shuffle his or her feet

D. avoid the use of assistive walking devices

51. A machine that is used to lift a patient from one place to another is called a:

A. wheelchair

B. mechanical lift

C. transfer bench

D. gait belt

52. Considerations for using a portable mechanical lift include:

A. removing the sling from behind the patient once the transfer is complete

B. transporting the patient from the bedroom to the living room recliner

C. attaching the hooks on the sling through the metal frame facing out away from the patient

D. all of the above

53. When helping a patient to stand, the first instruction the home care aide gives is:

A. "Put one foot in under you."

B. "Move to the front of your chair or bed."

C. "On the count of three, push down with your arms, lean forward, stand up."

D. "Put your hands around my waist."

54. When assisting a patient to sit, you should do all of the following except:
    A. be sure the wheels on the bed or wheel-chair are locked
    B. remind the patient to feel the bed or chair with the back of his or her legs
    C. direct the patient to sit down while holding onto your waist
    D. support and direct the activity as the patient sits down

55. When assisting a patient to go up stairs using a cane, remember the following:
    A. Advance the weakest leg to the next step.
    B. Advance the strongest leg to the next step.
    C. Advance the cane first.
    D. none of the above

56. Guidelines for using assistive walking devices include all of the following except:
    A. canes, crutches, and walkers must always be used with rubber tips on the ends
    B. screws and bolts should be securely in place
    C. wooden canes and crutches should be smooth without cracks
    D. pull up on walkers and canes to come to a standing position

57. When using crutches, the patient's body weight is placed on:
    A. the patient's hands and arms
    B. the patient's shoulders
    C. the patient's feet
    D. none of the above

58. Mr. Green has asked you to assist him to sit on the edge of the bed. The first thing you should do is:
    A. position your feet with a wide base of support and your center of gravity close to the bed
    B. tell Mr. Green what you are going to do
    C. roll Mr. Green onto his side facing you
    D. swing Mr. Green's legs over the edge of the bed

59. When assisting Mrs. Hall with crutch walking, you should instruct her to:
    A. place her weight on the top of her crutches
    B. place her crutches 8 to 12 inches in front of her body, then swing her body through
    C. adjust the crutches if they feel uncomfortable
    D. all of the above

60. When you assist your patient with a pivot transfer from bed to chair, the wheelchair should be placed:
    A. at the head of the bed
    B. at the foot of the bed
    C. at a 45 degree angle to the bed
    D. at the patient's involved side

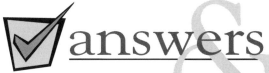

answers & rationales

1.

A. Placing the chair at a 45 degree angle to the bed helps to minimize the distance the patient must move, and transferring toward the stronger side gives the patient the best balance. *(Zucker, p. 245)*

2.

A. Your foot is placed near the patient's foot to prevent slipping or sliding. Your feet should be shoulder-width apart for good base of support during the transfer. *(Zucker, p.245)*

3.

B. Assist the patient to a sitting position before you place his or her hand on the arm of the chair for transfer. *(Zucker, p. 245)*

4.

C. Other terms may apply to specific types of walking or movement, but ambulation refers only to walking. *(Zucker, p. 246)*

5.

B. Standing on the patients's weak side and using a guarding belt will help you to have control if the patient starts to fall or grow weak. *(Zucker, p.246)*

6.

D. To prevent falls or other accidents, lock the wheels on the chair first, then perform the other steps in the procedure. *(Zucker, p. 246)*

7.

D. All of these are appropriate actions to take for safely assisting a patient with ambulation. *(Zucker, p. 246)*

8.

B. These steps are the safest and most effective way to help the patient who needs minimal assistance to move from sitting to standing. *(Zucker, p. 244)*

9.

A. Patients with a weak side should always move toward the stronger side to maintain balance, and placing the chair at a 45 degree angle to the bed helps to minimize the distance the patient must move. *(Zucker, p. 246)*

10.

C. By advancing the stronger leg first, then the crutch, and then the weaker leg, the patient remains balanced on the stronger leg and crutch while going up the stairs and is less likely to lose balance or fall. *(Zucker, p. 247)*

11.

A. By advancing the cane, then the weaker leg, then the stronger leg, the patient remains balanced on the strong leg and the cane while the weaker leg is advanced going down the stairs and is less likely to lose balance or fall. *(Zucker, p. 247)*

12.

C. Neither the walker nor the cane is secure enough for the patient to use it to pull up to a standing position. *(Zucker, p. 247)*

13.

C. This balances the patient's weight between the cane and the weaker side. *(Zucker, p. 247)*

14.

D. All of these steps are used to ambulate correctly using a cane. *(Zucker, p. 248)*

15.

A. The standard three-point gait allows the patient to balance weight on both crutches and then advance the stronger foot. *(Zucker, p. 249)*

16.

A. When you stand on the weaker side and a little behind the patient, you can support the patient if he or she begins to fall or loses his or her balance. *(Zucker, p. 246)*

17.

C. The physical therapist or nurse will teach the proper placement of devices and the gait to be used; the homemaker or home health aide is responsible for assisting the patient to use the device correctly and safely. *(Zucker, p. 246)*

18.

B. The walker should be picked up and moved when the patient's feet are stationary; then the feet should be moved while the walker is stationary to prevent loss of balance and falls. *(Zucker, p. 250)*

19.

C. The patient should let go of the assistive device and hold onto the arms of the chair as he or she lowers himself or herself into the chair. The assistive device is not stable enough to support the patient's weight while the patient lowers himself or herself into a chair. *(Zucker, p. 250)*

20.

D. All of these observations are important and should be recorded in the patient's chart. *(Zucker, p. 245)*

21.

D. All of these are reasons for using the same sequence of actions each time you assist a patient to stand. *(Zucker, p. 243)*

22.

D. All of these are environmental barriers in using adaptive equipment. *(Zucker, p. 234)*

23.

A. Using a wide base of support and keeping your load close to your center of gravity are basics in body mechanics. Avoid bending at the waist, and keep your weight distributed evenly between both feet. *(Zucker, p. 250)*

24.

C. Guarding belts are used to help you control the patient at his or her center of gravity if the patient loses his balance and begins to fall; they are not used to pull a patient. *(Zucker, p. 246)*

25.

C. A dining room chair with arm rests gives the patient good support and arms that he or she can use when sitting and standing. Recliners and soft-cushioned chairs are difficult for patients to get out of, and the patient's feet must rest on the floor for him or her to be able to get up safely. *(Zucker, p. 240)*

26.

D. All of these actions are appropriate to take when you are using a portable mechanical patient lift. *(Zucker, p. 242)*

27.

C. The sling is left in the chair under the patient so that when you are ready to move the patient back to bed, all you need to do is hook the lift to the sling. It would be difficult, if not impossible, to remove the sling from beneath a patient who is in a sitting position. *(Zucker, p.243)*

28.

A. The patient's legs are hanging down and must be guided by you so that they do not bump into objects or into the lift. *(Zucker, p. 243)*

29.

C. If you are unsure how to operate a piece of equipment, do not use the equipment. Call your supervisor for help. Do not depend on family members to show you how to do your job. *(Zucker, p. 250)*

30.

C. It is not appropriate for you to force a patient to use the cane by threats, refuse to care for him if he does not use it, or let him do as he pleases without attempting to explain and educate him. This is a safety issue, and your supervisor must be made aware of the situation. *(Zucker, p. 246)*

31.

D. To avoid a possible fall or loss of balance due to the patient's mental state, you should perform all of these interventions. *(Zucker, p. 242)*

32.

A. Whenever possible, you should prioritize your care according to patient and family wishes. You can be flexible in your work and do other things first, then get the patient up after she has had time to rest. *(Zucker, pp. 34–35)*

33.

B. You are negligent when you fail to give proper care when you know how to do so and the result is physical or emotional harm to the patient. *(Zucker, p. 13)*

34.

C. Do not make changes in the way the patient has been taught to use assistive equipment. This is the role of the nurse or physical therapist. Reporting the family and patient's concerns to your supervisor will help the issue to be reviewed and revised as needed. *(Zucker, p. 246)*

35.

C. Requests for assistive equipment should be handled through your supervisor. *(Zucker, p. 246)*

36.

A. The patient must turn, or pivot, to move from the chair to the bed. He or she cannot transfer by bending, stretching, or stepping up. *(Zucker, p. 245)*

37.

B. A guarding belt (transfer belt) can help to give you better control over the patient's center of gravity when assisting with ambulation. *(Zucker, p. 240)*

38.

D. Utilize your patient's existing abilities, especially when transferring—for your safety and for the patient's safety. *(Zucker, p. 245)*

39.

C. Safety—for yourself and the patient—is a key principle in any patient care activity, especially with transfers or moving patients. *(Zucker, p. 240)*

40.

A. A guarding (transfer) belt is buckled around the patient's midsection and over the patient's clothing. *(Zucker, p. 240)*

41.

A. Support the patient's weak side, permitting the patient to freely use his or her strong side and assist with the transfer. *(Zucker, pp. 182, 245)*

42.

C. The chair should provide good support to the patient's back. *(Zucker, p. 240)*

43.

D. A mechanical lift is used to transfer a patient; the other devices are used to assist with ambulation. *(Zucker, pp. 246–247)*

44.

D. The cane is usually used on the stronger side. That way, the patient's weight will be balanced between the cane and the involved (weak) side. *(Zucker, pp. 247–248)*

45.

C. A guarding (transfer) belt helps you to maintain control over the patient's center of gravity and provides a safety measure for you and the patient. *(Zucker, p. 240)*

46.

D. Hand washing should be performed before and after the transfer (and any other patient care procedure). *(Zucker, p. 245)*

47.

A. This is a change from what would be considered normal and must be reported. *(Zucker, p. 241)*

48.

A. One of the primary functions of the physical therapist is to assist with activities of motion, such as transfers and ambulation. *(Zucker, p. 234)*

49.

D. A walker provides support and safety for a patient because of imbalance or weakness. It offers more support than a cane. *(Zucker, p. 250)*

50.

A. Standing on the patient's weaker side and slightly behind him or her gives you a position of safety for both you and the patient. *(Zucker, pp. 246–247)*

51.

B. A mechanical lift is used to transfer patients who are too weak and/or too heavy to be transferred by a person. *(Zucker, p. 242)*

52.

C. Attach the sling to the mechanical lift with the hooks in place through the metal frame facing outward to avoid scraping the patient's skin. *(Zucker, p. 243)*

53.

B. The sequence begins with instructing the patient to "move to the front of the chair or bed." This gets the patient closer to you for safety and proper body mechanics for both of you. *(Zucker, p. 244)*

54.

C. You should direct the patient to reach back for the arms of the chair or the surface of the bed to provide support for himself or herself and maintain proper body mechanics for you. *(Zucker, p. 244)*

55.

B. Advance the strongest leg to the next step before bringing the cane forward, and then move the weaker leg to the next step. *(Zucker, p. 247)*

56.

D. Do *not* come to a standing position pulling up walkers or canes. They are not stable. *(Zucker, p. 247)*

57.

A. The body's weight is on the hands and arms, not on the top of the crutch under the arms. *(Zucker, pp. 248–249)*

58.

B. Inform the patient what you intend to do, how you intend to do it, and how he or she can assist. *(Zucker, p. 241)*

59.

B. Her weight should be on her arms and hands. Never adjust the crutches; the physical therapist will do that as needed. Crutches should be placed 8 to 12 inches in front of the body before moving forward. *(Zucker, p. 249)*

60.

C. The wheelchair should be placed at a 45 degree angle to the bed so that the patient will move toward his stronger side. *(Zucker, p. 245)*

14 Range of Motion and Positioning

chapter objectives

Upon completion of Chapter 14, the student is responsible for the following:

➤ Define principles of range-of-motion exercises.

➤ Describe basics of good skin care.

➤ Identify risks of skin breakdown.

➤ Describe effects of aging on the skin.

➤ Identify pressure points to body areas.

➤ Define bedsores (decubitus ulcers).

➤ Describe bed positioning.

DIRECTIONS
Each of the questions or incomplete statements below is followed by four suggested answers or completions. Select **one answer** that is best in each case.

1. When a person has restricted movement, joint motion may become painful and limited. This is because of the:
   A. shortening and tightening of muscles
   B. calcification of the tendons and joints
   C. inflammation of the muscles and joints
   D. atrophy of the joints

2. When a patient is unable to move an extremity, a caregiver can exercise it for him or her. This is called:
   A. active range of motion
   B. passive range of motion
   C. assistive daily activities
   D. daily range of motion

3. When assisting a patient to do range of motion with his or her neck, your hands should be:
   A. under the patient's chin, one on each side
   B. around the patient's neck providing support at the back
   C. on the patient's forehead with your fingers locked together
   D. over the patient's ears with your fingers toward the face

4. Daily range of motion performed by the patient will:
   A. keep the muscles flexible
   B. maintain joint movement
   C. strengthen muscles
   D. all of the above

5. When a patient performs his or her own prescribed exercises, this is called:
   A. active range of motion
   B. passive range of motion
   C. self-motion
   D. limited support motion

6. The type of health professional who will set up the necessary range of motion exercises for the patient is a/an:
   A. occupational therapist
   B. range of motion therapist
   C. physical therapist
   D. physician

7. Rehabilitation is best defined as:
   A. receiving physical therapy to cure a disability
   B. the use of braces and other devices for walking
   C. the process of relearning how to function
   D. returning the patient to self-care

8. Which of the following statements is *not* true about muscles?
   A. They shorten and tighten if not used.
   B. Resistive range of motion increases muscle strength.
   C. Muscles move bones.
   D. Pain must be endured if exercise is to strengthen muscles.

9. Principles of good body mechanics include:
   A. supporting a joint when doing range of motion on a patient
   B. stretch a muscle, let it rest, and then stretch it again
   C. stand a full arm's length from the patient when doing range of motion
   D. all of the above

10. In assisting the patient with range of motion, it is best to:
   A. expect the patient to do as much as possible
   B. work at the patient's level and speed

C. use resistive range of motion to increase muscle strength

D. all of the above

11. Which of the following terms is used to refer to the body part or side that is affected by the patient's disease or injury?

A. functional

B. involved

C. diseased

D. handicapped

12. If the patient experiences pain while receiving range-of-motion exercises, you should:

A. accept the complaint as a warning sign, stop, and notify your supervisor

B. explain that without pain, there will be no strengthening and continue

C. use hot packs on the painful area about 20 minutes before the next exercise

D. call the physical therapist and report the pain

13. Which of the following is *not* true about range-of-motion exercises?

A. Never bend or straighten a body part farther than it will go.

B. Slow, steady movement of a muscle will help it to relax and increase the joint range.

C. Use only the flat part of your hand and fingers to grip the patient's body parts.

D. Do not perform range of motion on a forgetful patient.

14. The proper way to do shoulder flexion is to:

A. keep the arm at shoulder level, reach across the chest past the opposite shoulder, then reach out to the side

B. with the elbow straight, raise the arm over the head, then lower the arm, keeping it in front of you the whole time

C. with the elbow straight, raise the arm over the head, then lower the arm, keeping it out to the side the whole time

D. with the arm alongside the body, bend the elbow to touch the shoulder, then straighten the elbow out again

15. To perform shoulder horizontal abduction and adduction, you should:

A. keep the arm at shoulder level, reach across the chest past the opposite shoulder, then reach out to the side

B. with the elbow straight, raise the arm over the head, then lower the arm, keeping it in front of you the whole time

C. with the elbow straight, raise the arm over the head, then lower the arm, keeping it out to the side the whole time

D. with the arm alongside the body, bend the elbow to touch the shoulder, then straighten the elbow out again

16. Which of the following is an example of adduction and abduction?

A. Make a fist, then straighten the fingers out together.

B. Touch the thumb to the tip of each finger to make a circle. Open the hand fully between touching each finger.

C. With the fingers straight, squeeze the fingers together, then spread them apart.

D. Touch the tip of each finger to its base, then straighten each finger in turn.

17. Which of the following is an example of finger/thumb opposition?

A. Make a fist, then straighten the fingers out together.

B. Touch the thumb to the tip of each finger to make a circle. Open the hand fully between touching each finger.

C. With the fingers straight, squeeze the fingers together, then spread them apart.

D. Touch the tip of each finger to its base, then straighten each finger in turn.

18. Which of the following is an example of forearm pronation and supination?
    A. With the arm alongside the body and the elbow bent to 90 degrees, turn the forearm so that the palm faces first toward the head, then toward the feet.
    B. With the arm out straight from the body, bend the wrist back and forth and in a circle.
    C. With the arm alongside the body, bend the elbow in a right angle and move the forearm from side to side and up and down.
    D. With the arm alongside the body and flat on the bed, lift the forearm up from the elbow and then push the palm down on the bed.

19. Which of the following is an example of a quad set?
    A. With legs flat on the bed, tighten thigh muscles to straighten the knee, pushing the thigh into the bed, hold for a count of five, then relax.
    B. With one knee bent and the foot flat on the bed, turn the leg so that the knee moves out to the side, then inward across the other leg.
    C. Keeping the knee straight, raise the leg up off the bed, then return it slowly to the bed.
    D. With legs flat on the bed and feet apart, turn both legs so that the knees face outward, then turn so that the knees face each other.

20. Bending the ankles up, down, and from side to side is an example of:
    A. abduction and flexion
    B. abduction and adduction
    C. pronation and extension
    D. dorsiflexion and extension

21. Bending and straightening the toes is an example of:
    A. abduction and flexion
    B. abduction and adduction

C. internal and external rotation
D. flexion and extension

22. Which of the following is an example of hip and knee flexion and extension?
    A. Bend the knee and bring it up toward the chest, keeping the foot off the bed; lower the leg to bed, straightening the knee as it goes down.
    B. With the leg flat on the bed and the knee pointing to the ceiling, slide the leg out to the side, then slide it back to touch the other leg.
    C. Keeping the knee straight, raise the leg up off the bed, then return it slowly to the bed with the knee straight.
    D. With both knees bent up, feet flat on the bed, push on the bed with the feet to raise the hips, hold for a count of five, then relax.

23. Which of the following is an example of bridging?
    A. Bend the knee and bring it up toward the chest, keeping the foot off the bed; lower the leg to bed, straightening the knee as it goes down.
    B. With the leg flat on the bed and the knee pointing to the ceiling, slide the leg out to the side, then slide it back to touch the other leg.
    C. Keeping the knee straight, raise the leg up off the bed, then return it slowly to the bed with the knee straight.
    D. With both knees bent up, feet flat on the bed, push on the bed with the feet to raise the hips, hold for a count of five, then relax.

24. Bending the toes is an example of:
    A. adduction
    B. abduction
    C. flexion
    D. extension

25. Which of the following will ensure that the patient receives maximum benefit from range-of-motion exercises?
    A. Include the family in the exercises so that they can give them when you are not there.
    B. Follow a logical sequence during the exercises so that each joint and muscle is exercised.
    C. Report to your supervisor if the exercises are getting harder for the patient to do, rather than easier.
    D. all of the above

26. Body alignment refers to the:
    A. body shape type of the patient
    B. position of the body in relation to the bed or chair
    C. arrangement of the body in a straight line with body parts in correct anatomical position
    D. position of the spine in relation to the head

27. When positioning a patient, it is important to prevent shearing. Ways to do this include:
    A. using a pull sheet to position the patient
    B. protecting bony prominences with sheepskin or egg-crate padding
    C. having the patient do as much of the moving as possible
    D. all of the above

28. General positioning rules include which of the following?
    A. The hand on the involved side should be positioned open with the palm flat.
    B. A swollen limb should be positioned higher than the heart.
    C. Pressure sores will heal more quickly if bandaged.
    D. all of the above.

29. In talking to the patient, which of the following terms is used to refer to the body part or side that is affected by injury or disease?
    A. handicapped
    B. nonfunctional
    C. involved
    D. disabled

30. When positioning the patient on his or her back, you should:
    A. place a folded bath towel under the hip of the involved side
    B. place a small pillow under the calf of the weak leg with the heel hanging off the edge of the mattress
    C. support the feet with the bottom of the feet and toes at a 90 degree angle to the bed
    D. all of the above

31. When the patient is lying on his or her back, you should:
    A. place a rolled washcloth in the hand on the uninvolved side
    B. place a small folded towel under the shoulderblade of the involved side
    C. use pillows under the legs and knees for support
    D. all of the above

32. When positioning a patient on his or her uninvolved side, you should:
    A. place a pillow between the patient's knees
    B. place a pillow under both arms so that they are level with the shoulders
    C. place a rolled washcloth in the uninvolved hand
    D. all of the above

33. The major difference between positioning the patient on the involved side and positioning on the uninvolved side is that while on the involved side:
    A. the patient's comfort will be the key to how and where support is used
    B. the patient's position will need to be changed more frequently
    C. the involved side must be checked more frequently for signs of pressure and skin irritation
    D. all of the above

34. Each time the position of the bedfast patient is changed, you must:
   A. check the bony prominences for redness
   B. bathe the side which the patient has been lying on
   C. apply powder and cornstarch to the sheets
   D. all of the above

35. In helping a patient to move up in bed, one method of preventing strain on the patient and yourself is to:
   A. tell the patient what to do and let him or her do it
   B. use a counting signal for movement, such as "one, two, three"
   C. raise the head of the bed to a near sitting position
   D. all of the above

36. When moving a patient up in bed with his or her help, you should stand:
   A. with your feet 12 inches apart
   B. with your foot that is closest to the head of the bed pointed in that direction
   C. with your knees bent and your back straight
   D. all of the above

37. Which of the following would *not* be correct in helping a patient to raise his or her head and shoulders from the bed?
   A. holding your arm out steady, position your feet, and allow the patient to pull up on you
   B. with your feet 12 inches apart, bending your knees, grasping the patient's shoulders, and pulling him or her up
   C. grasping the patient by the wrists and pulling to lift his or her head and shoulders from the bed
   D. all of the above

38. When assisting a patient to move up in bed, your hands should be:
   A. one under the patient's shoulder and the other under his or her knees

   B. one under the small of his back and the other under his or her neck
   C. one under the patient's shoulder and the other under the patient's buttocks
   D. one under the patient's shoulder closest to you and the other under the patient's armpit on the opposite side

39. When two people are moving the patient up in bed, you should:
   A. roll the drawsheet up to the patient's body and grab underhand
   B. stand so that you are slightly turned toward the head of the bed
   C. shift the weight of your body from your back leg to your front leg as you move
   D. all of the above

40. In positioning the patient in bed, it is best to always:
   A. move the pillow out from under the patient's head
   B. keep your feet together and your arms bent
   C. raise the head of the bed to its highest position
   D. all of the above

41. When the patient cannot assist you to move him or her up in bed, you could:
   A. grasp the pull sheet and move one side of the patient up then go to the other side and repeat the process until the patient is at the head of the bed
   B. place one arm under the patient's shoulders and the other under his or her knees and lift the patient up
   C. stand at the head of the bed, grasp the top of the pull sheet, shift your weight to your back leg, and slide the patient to the top of the bed
   D. all of the above

42. Which of the following activities are done when moving the patient in any way?

A. removing the top sheet to prevent restriction of movement

B. raising the head of the bed to a comfortable height

C. locking the wheels on the bed or securing it

D. all of the above

43. When a bedfast patient is lying on his or her back, he or she should be:

A. on one side of the bed so that when turned to his or her side, the patient will be in the center of the bed

B. placed in the center of the bed so that he or she can next be turned to either side

C. lying with his or her head elevated at least 45 degrees

D. lying flat with a towel roll under his or her neck

44. Which of the following should be done first in positioning a helpless patient on his or her back?

A. Slide both arms under the patient's buttocks and slide them toward you.

B. Slide both arms under the patient's feet and slide them toward you.

C. Slide both arms under the patient's back to the far shoulder and slide the shoulders toward you.

D. Comfortably position the head.

45. When you log roll the patient toward you, your hands should be:

A. placed gently, one behind the patient's neck and one behind his or her knees

B. both placed in the small of the patient's back for support

C. holding the patient at his or her hip and shoulder

D. one under the armpit on the opposite side with the patient's arm over yours and one in the bend of his knees

46. Methods to keep the bedfast patient safe when no rails are present include:

A. placing a dining room chair next to the bed

B. having tissues and other needed items within short reach

C. devising a method for the patient to signal for someone

D. all of the above

47. Which statement is *not* true about skin care for the patient?

A. Good skin care is a primary responsibility of the homemaker or home health aide.

B. Damaged or broken skin is the fault of the homemaker or home health aide.

C. Disease processes and poor nutrition contribute to the condition of the patient's skin.

D. Medications and mobility can directly affect the condition of the patient's skin.

48. Observations of the skin on a daily basis include:

A. temperature and color

B. comparison of extremities

C. cleanliness and dryness

D. all of the above

49. A bruise can be the result of:

A. a reaction to a medication

B. a change in diet

C. a change in a patient's ability to perform some task

D. all of the above

50. More problems are encountered with the skin of the elderly because:

A. of a loss of skin tone

B. of an increase in the fatty layer under the skin

C. the enlarged veins provide too much circulation

D. all of the above

51. The reason that bony prominences such as the shoulderblades, elbows, heels, and backbone are more prone to decubitus formation is that:
    A. there is more loss of skin tone in these areas as we age
    B. they are covered by thin layers of skin that receive a smaller blood supply than other areas
    C. these areas are more prone to loss of natural oils as we age, decreasing the flexibility of the skin
    D. all of the above

52. Documentation of bruises or reddened areas of the skin includes:
    A. any changes in size or color from day to day
    B. any changes in the patient's appitite
    C. any arguments or upsetting events in the patient's day
    D. all of the above

53. Basic skin care for an elderly patient should include:
    A. washing and changing an incontinent patient so that he or she is always clean
    B. a complete bath or shower every day
    C. use of antiperspirants and perfumes daily
    D. all of the above

54. The best way to help the elderly patient with dry skin is to:
    A. use bath salts daily
    B. never use soap
    C. vigorously rub the skin to remove dry skin which will prevent itching
    D. none of the above

55. A major concern in protecting the skin of the elderly is:
    A. bruises can be unsightly and cause depression
    B. an adequate diet is necessary to prevent wrinkling

C. scratching can introduce bacteria and lead to infection
    D. all of the above

56. Factors that increase the chances of damage to the skin of the elderly include:
    A. incontinence
    B. lying on the catheter or other types of tubing
    C. decreased movement
    D. all of the above

57. Negligence is a legal term. The home care aide can be found guilty of negligence for:
    A. failure to turn a bedfast patient every 2 hours while on duty
    B. failure to give a tub bath to a patient every day
    C. arguing with a family member
    D. all of the above

58. Patients who are bedbound are at greatest risk for:
    A. stiff joints
    B. bedsores
    C. bladder infections
    D. decreased appetite

59. Mr. Carter has diabetes. In providing his foot care, the home care aide should consider which of the following?
    A. Cutting toenails is permissible if requested.
    B. Feet should be soaked in water and bath oil for 5 minutes every day.
    C. Advise him to wear well-fitting shoes when out of bed.
    D. Dry, cracked skin is acceptable.

60. While you are providing skin care for Ms. Bell, she asks you to rub her back "real hard." You should:
    A. avoid rubbing the skin hard
    B. rub her back with alcohol

C. rub her back and scratch

D. use a back scratcher

61. Places where obese patients are more prone
to bedsores include:

A. the outer thigh

B. under the breasts

C. the toes

D. the earlobes

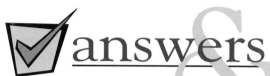
1.

A. When muscles are not used, they shorten and tighten, which limits motion and may cause pain with motion. *(Zucker, p. 234)*

2.

B. "Passive" indicates range-of-motion exercises during which the patient does not help. *(Zucker, p. 236)*

3.

D. To move the neck through its full range of motion, the hands must be placed on either side of the head. *(Zucker, p. 235)*

4.

D. All of these are benefits of daily range-of-motion exercise. *(Zucker, p. 234)*

5.

A. Active range of motion is done totally by the patient. *(Zucker, p. 236)*

6.

C. The physical therapist reviews the whole patient profile, including the environment, when setting up a routine. Occupational therapists work with patients on activities of daily living, not exercises for joint and muscle flexibility. *(Zucker, p. 233)*

7.

C. Rehabilitation does not necessarily return a patient to self-care, nor does it cure a disability. Rehabilitation may involve many types of assistive and adaptive devices to help the patient relearn how to function. *(Zucker, p. 233)*

8.

D. Pain is a warning sign and should be heeded. Never take a patient beyond the point of pain. *(Zucker, p. 236)*

9.

A. Joints must be supported during range of motion to prevent strain *(Zucker, p. 237)*

10.

D. All of these guidelines are appropriate to use in assisting patients with range-of-motion exercises. *(Zucker, pp. 234–236)*

11.

B. "Diseased" and "handicapped" are words that have negative connotations. A functional body part is one that works correctly. An involved body part is one that has been affected by disease or injury. *(Zucker, p. 182)*

12.

A. Pain is a warning sign and should be heeded. It is not necessary for patients to experience pain to receive benefits from range-of-motion exercises. Your supervisor should be notified and can communicate with the physical therapist about the problem. *(Zucker, p. 236)*

13.

D. Even if the person does not appear to understand, the tone of your voice and the touch of your hands help to communicate. *(Zucker, p. 236)*

14.

B. The shoulder is flexed only when the arm is moved over the head and back to the side with the elbow straight. Other options flex or extend other joints. *(Zucker, p. 237)*

15.

A. The shoulder is abducted and adducted horizontally with this motion; other options flex or extend other joints. *(Zucker, p. 237)*

16.

C. Fingers abduct and adduct with this motion; other options exercise fingers in different ways than abduction and adduction. *(Zucker, p. 238)*

17.

B. This is a description of exercising finger/thumb opposition; other options exercise fingers in other ways. *(Zucker, p. 238)*

18.

A. This motion turns the arm from supination to pronation; other options exercise the arm in different ways. *(Zucker, p. 238)*

19.

A. Quadriceps muscles are those in the anterior upper thigh, so tightening and relaxing this area will flex the quadriceps muscles. *(Zucker, p. 239)*

20.

D. Bending ankles up dorsiflexes and bending them down extends the muscles in the ankles. *(Zucker, p. 239)*

21.

D. Flexion refers to bending the toes, and extension refers to straightening the toes. *(Zucker, p. 239)*

22.

A. This motion bends and straightens the hip and knee. Other options exercise the hip and knee in different ways. *(Zucker, p. 238)*

23.

D. This exercise lifts the hips off the bed, causing the body to form a "bridge." Other options exercise the legs in different ways. *(Zucker, p. 239)*

24.

C. To flex means to bend a joint. *(Zucker, p. 239)*

25.

D. All of these actions will help the patient to recieve maximum benefit from range-of-motion exercises. *(Zucker, p. 236)*

26.

C. Alignment refers to the straightness of the body. Correct anatomical position is necessary for all parts of the body to be in the right place to prevent contractures or other problems. *(Zucker, p. 182)*

27.

D. All of these are ways to prevent shearing while moving and positioning patients. *(Zucker, p. 193)*

28.

B. Positioning a swollen limb higher than the heart allows gravity to help drain the extra fluid from the limb. *(Zucker, p. 183)*

29.

C. The body part or side that is affected by injury or disease is involved in treatment, so it is referred to as the involved side. *(Zucker, p. 182)*

30.

D. All of these actions should be taken when you position a patient on his or her back to promote good body alignment and patient comfort. *(Zucker, p. 183)*

31.

B. Placing a small folded towel under the shoulderblade of the involved side will make it easier and more comfortable to elevate the arm and elbow on a pillow higher than the heart *(Zucker, p. 183)*

32.

A. A pillow placed between the patient's knees helps to keep the hips and low back in proper body alignment; it also prevents pressure areas from developing where the legs rest against one another. *(Zucker, p. 184)*

33.

D. All of these guidelines apply in positioning the patient on his involved side. *(Zucker, p. 184)*

34.

A. Bony prominences become reddened quickly and can easily deteriorate into decubitus ulcers. You will detect any problems as early as possible by checking each time you change the patient's position. *(Zucker p. 197)*

35.

B. When you and the patient move at the same time, such as on the count of three, you decrease pull and resistance during movement. This helps you to use better body mechanics, and helps to prevent shear and friction for your patient. *(Zucker, p. 185)*

36.

D. All of these actions demonstrate the use of good body mechanics. *(Zucker, p. 185)*

37.

C. Grasping the patient by the wrists and pulling can dislocate or subluxate the patient's shoulder. It is best to let the patient pull up on you. *(Zucker, p. 189)*

38.

C. You help move the patient's center of gravity, his or her heaviest part, when you place your hands in this manner. *(Zucker, p. 185)*

39.

D. All of these are actions to take when two people move the patient up in bed. *(Zucker, p. 186)*

40.

A. Removing the pillow from under the patient's head allows you to move him or her up on a level surface. Keeping the bed as flat as possible helps you to move the patient up with less effort. *(Zucker, p. 187)*

41.

C. You use good body mechanics when you pull the patient toward you. When you stand at the head of the bed and pull, you move the patient up in bed without trying to push or lift him or her. *(Zucker, p. 187)*

42.

C. The bed must be locked or secured to keep it from rolling or moving away from you when you are moving the patient. *(Zucker, pp. 185–188)*

43.

A. If a patient is not moved to the side of the bed before being turned in the opposite direction, he or she may end up wedged against the side rails when turned. *(Zucker, p. 188)*

44.

C. Move the shoulders toward you first to prevent twisting the trunk of the patient's body. *(Zucker, p. 188)*

45.

C. Placing your hands in this fashion helps you to roll the patient as a unit, without allowing his or her back to twist *(Zucker, p. 189)*

46.

D. All of these actions help to keep the bedfast patient safe when no rails are present *(Zucker, p. 138)*

47.

B. Often, even with good practices, patients suffer from skin breakdown. It is important for you to know that you have done all you can to prevent skin breakdown. *(Zucker, p. 198)*

48.

D. All of these observations should be made daily because they give information about the patient's overall health. *(Zucker, p. 193)*

49.

D. Any of these situations can cause a bruise. *(Zucker, p. 193)*

50.

A. Aging causes a gradual loss of skin tone, including drying of natural oils and loss of the layer of fat under the skin. *(Zucker, p. 193)*

51.

B. Areas that are covered by thin skin layers receive a smaller blood supply and are more suseptible to pressure and skin breakdown. *(Zucker, p. 193)*

52.

A. Changes in size and color of bruises and reddened areas give information about the patient's condition and healing status. *(Zucker, p. 193)*

53.

A. Keeping the patient dry and clean helps to prevent infections and skin breakdown. A complete bath or shower is not necessary every day and may dry skin. Antiperspirants and perfumes may dry the skin or cause skin reactions. *(Zucker, p. 195)*

54.

D. None of these actions is appropriate when caring for elderly patients with dry skin. *(Zucker, pp. 195–196)*

55.

C. The skin is the body's first line of defense against infection; when the skin is broken bacteria can enter the body. *(Zucker, p. 195)*

56.

D. All of these factors increase skin damage in the elderly. *(Zucker, p. 196)*

57.

A. Negligence means failing to give proper care. Bedfast patients must be turned every 2 hours to prevent skin breakdown. *(Zucker, p. 13)*

58.

B. Bedsores, or pressure sores, are areas where the skin has broken because of pressure. Bedbound patients are at great risk for bedsores. *(Zucker, p. 197)*

59.

C. The proper shoes are well fitting and give support. Going barefooted is not advised. *(Zucker, p. 199)*

60.

A. Hard rubbing can damage skin that is fragile. Always rub the skin with lotion and in a circular motion. *(Zucker, p. 196)*

61.

B. Obese patients tend to develop bedsores where body parts rub together, causing friction, such as under the breasts, between the folds of the buttocks, and between the thighs. *(Zucker, p. 197)*

15 Medications

chapter objectives

Upon completion of Chapter 15, the student is responsible for the following:

➤ Describe medication issues among the elderly.

➤ Describe medication assistance for the home care aide.

➤ Identify techniques for assisting patients with medications.

➤ Describe medication storage and disposal.

➤ Describe oxygen use and safety.

DIRECTIONS
Each of the questions or incomplete statements below is followed by four suggested answers or completions. Select **one answer** that is best in each case.

1. The responsibility of the home care aide when the patient is to take medication is to:
   A. remind the patient that it is time to take the medication
   B. put the pill in the patient's hand
   C. instruct the family to help if needed
   D. all of the above

2. If the patient needs assistance with taking medication, you can:
   A. loosen the bottle caps
   B. hold the patient's hand to help steady the glass of water
   C. place the medication bottles within reach of the patient
   D. all of the above

3. Your patient is to receive eye drops four times a day. If necessary, you can:
   A. hold the eyelids open as you drop the medication into the eye
   B. wipe any excess liquid from under the eye, wiping from the nose outward
   C. place your hand on the patient's forehead to tilt the head backward so that you will not spill the drops
   D. all of the above

4. Which of the following might indicate a reaction to a medication?
   A. difficulty breathing
   B. rash, itching
   C. diarrhea
   D. all of the above

5. If your patient starts vomiting shortly after taking a medication, you should:
   A. notify your supervisor
   B. have the patient repeat the medication

   C. have the family call the doctor for something for nausea
   D. all of the above

6. When you place the patient's medications in front of him, he spends a long time reading the labels of each one. You should:
   A. encourage the patient to hurry so that the medication will be taken on time
   B. tell the patient that his family will have to start giving him his medication if he is going to be so slow
   C. tell the patient that you have already checked each of the labels
   D. allow the patient to read each of the labels

7. Your patient feels nauseated and does not want to take her blood pressure pill. You should:
   A. check her blood pressure to see whether she needs it
   B. notify your supervisor
   C. give her the pill with a cracker and soda
   D. all of the above

8. Your responsibility after the patient has taken medications is to:
   A. check that the caps are tight on the bottles
   B. chart the time and how the medication was taken
   C. place the medications where the patient wants them kept
   D. all of the above

9. Which of the following is *not* one of the five rights of medication?
   A. The patient has a right to adjust dosages on the basis of his or her pain level.
   B. The medication must be for this patient.
   C. The correct medication for the patient at the right time.
   D. The correct dosage taken the right way.

10. Safety factors in the storage of medications include all of the following except:
    A. the practice of saving medications to treat the same symptoms in the future
    B. having separate storage places for medications with similar names
    C. not changing the storage location of medications without patient's permission
    D. store medications for different family members in separate places

11. Elderly patients:
    A. react to medications the same as younger patients do
    B. react to medications differently than younger patients do
    C. have no side effects to medications
    D. none of the above

12. Reasons elderly patients may stop taking medications include all of the following except:
    A. cost
    B. forgetfulness
    C. they like to be sick
    D. something they read about the drug

13. Your patient has been saving medications for many years, and they are in her top dresser drawer. You should:
    A. throw all the pills away
    B. burn all the medications
    C. notify your supervisor
    D. encourage the patient to return them for a refund

14. Your patient likes to take his wife's prescribed sleeping pills at night. The home care aide should:
    A. encourage him to take it with warm milk
    B. report this to the nurse supervisor
    C. loosen the lid so that it's not so hard for him to open
    D. notify the pharmacy of needed refills

15. Mrs. Smith is being treated for a urinary tract infection with an antibiotic. While assisting with her bath today, you notice a rash on her chest. You should:
    A. ask her whether it itches
    B. apply medicated lotion
    C. report this to your supervisor
    D. rub the rash area

16. Timmy is an 8-year-old boy for whom you provide care. Evidence of a medication reaction would be:
    A. difficulty breathing
    B. vomiting
    C. rash
    D. all of the above

17. Medications that are used to treat cancer are called:
    A. antibiotics
    B. chemotherapy
    C. radiation
    D. anti-inflammatory

18. Common skin reactions to chemotherapy include all of the following except:
    A. dry mouth and throat
    B. hair loss
    C. skin rashes
    D. pink nails

19. Checking the name of the medication with the list of medications left by the nurse is assuring which right of medications?
    A. the right patient
    B. the right medication
    C. the right time
    D. the right amount

20. Individuals who are licensed to administer medications include all of the following except:
    A. home care aide
    B. physician
    C. licensed practical nurse
    D. registered nurse

21. If the home care aide administers medications:
    A. the patient will feel better with a familiar face
    B. he or she takes all the responsibility for medications
    C. he or she should call the pharmacist
    D. he or she can give over-the-counter medications

22. Which of the following observations about medications should the home care aide report?
    A. The patient takes the medication on schedule.
    B. The patient does not know why he is taking his medications.
    C. The patient feels better after he takes his pain medication.
    D. The patient's indigestion goes away after taking his antacid.

23. All of the following should be reported after your patient takes a medication except:
    A. nausea
    B. itching
    C. difficulty breathing
    D. intact skin

24. When assisting the patient with medications, the home care aide may:
    A. loosen the tops of bottles or tubes
    B. squirt eye drops into the patient's eyes
    C. put ear drops into the patient's ears
    D. pour out pills from the bottle

25. A patient asks the home care aide to get her medication because her husband left it in another room. The home care aide should:
    A. obtain the bottle as requested
    B. obtain the bottle and pour out the correct amount
    C. tell the patient that she will have to wait until her husband returns
    D. call the physician

26. Medications that look alike should be:
    A. stored together
    B. combined into one bottle
    C. stored separately
    D. thrown out

27. Your supervisor has asked you to assist your patient to dispose of old medications. Considerations include all of the following except:
    A. flushing it down the toilet
    B. pouring it down a drain
    C. throwing it away in the garbage
    D. cutting up old medication patches

28. All of the following are considered medications except:
    A. oxygen
    B. aspirin
    C. Gatorade
    D. Tylenol

29. Information located on the medicine label includes all of the following except:
    A. name of medication
    B. name of patient
    C. name of home care agency
    D. name of physician

30. Putting a pill into a patient's mouth is considered:
    A. administering the medication
    B. assisting with the medication
    C. dosing the medication
    D. none of the above

31. A side effect of aspirin includes:
    A. bleeding
    B. improved appetite
    C. urination
    D. sweating

32. Your patient refuses to take her own medications. The home care aide should:
    A. pour out the pills and set them in front of her
    B. gently encourage her to take her pills
    C. call the physician
    D. call the pharmacy

33. The home care aide may assist with medications. This include all of the following except:
    A. observing when the patient takes the medication
    B. giving the medication
    C. recording observations
    D. reporting any problems to the supervisor

34. If more than one person in the house is taking the same medication:
    A. keep the medications together so that everyone will know where they are
    B. share the medications to keep down the cost
    C. keep the medications in separate places
    D. none of the above

35. Significant telephone numbers to be posted by the phone include all of the following except:
    A. family members
    B. poison control centers
    C. doctor
    D. the home care aide's home number

36. Drug misuse occurs when:
    A. a drug is taken too frequently
    B. patients double the amount to be taken

C. the drug is used by a person not under a doctor's orders
D. all of the above

37. Behaviors of drug dependency include all of the following except:
    A. reporting to work every day on time
    B. being secretive
    C. abusiveness
    D. extreme mood swings

38. Oxygen precautions include all of the following except:
    A. using a humidifier to help reduce static electricity
    B. using petroleum jelly on the patient's lips
    C. using oxygen tanks in cool areas
    D. placing "no smoking" signs inside and outside the patient's room

39. The health professional who dispenses medication is the:
    A. home care aide
    B. physician
    C. nurse
    D. pharmacist

40. Medications that can be purchased without a prescription are called:
    A. regular
    B. over-the-counter
    C. around-the-clock
    D. antibiotics

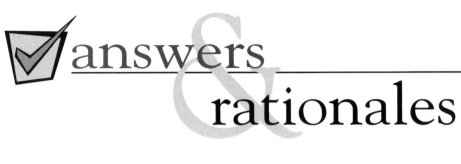

answers & rationales

1.

A. The home care aide assists the patient to take his or her own medication but does not administer the medication. *(Zucker, p.319)*

2.

D. All of these actions are forms of assisting a patient with his or her own medications, not administering medications. *(Zucker, p. 321)*

3.

B. This action is appropriate to assist the patient in administering his or her own eye drops. The other choices involve the home care aide administering the medication, which is not appropriate. *(Zucker, p. 321)*

4.

D. All of these can indicate some type of medication reaction, from mild to severe. *(Zucker, p. 320)*

5.

A. The patient may be reacting to the medication, so your supervisor must be notified. It is not in your role to repeat the medication or have the family obtain something for nausea. *(Zucker, p.320)*

6.

D. The label on the medication bottle must be checked every time the patient takes the medication. Because the patient administers the medication to himself, he should be sure he knows what medication he is obtaining. Do not rush medication preparation. *(Zucker, p. 321)*

7.

B. Medications are ordered by the physician. If the orders are not followed, the physician must be made aware of that fact. Your supervisor will take care of troubleshooting the problem and notifying the physician as necessary. *(Zucker, p. 319)*

8.

D. All of these are your responsibilities after the patient takes his or her medication. *(Zucker, p. 321)*

9.

A. Dosages of pain medication are ordered by the physician. It is not a patient right to adjust these doses. The physician can change the orders to accommodate the patient's needs. *(Zucker, p. 320)*

10.

A. The same symptoms can be caused by different physical problems. The practice of saving medication is most dangerous. Some medications change in chemical makeup as they age. *(Zucker, p. 321)*

11.

B. The older body reacts to and processes medications very differently from the younger body. *(Zucker, p. 61)*

12.

C. This is a myth—no one really likes to be sick. The elderly may stop taking medications for financial reasons, forgetfulness, or because they read or hear some news about the drug. *(Zucker, p. 61)*

13.

C. Some elderly patients save medications that become outdated and then start taking them again. The home care aide can help to maintain safe medication practice by notifying the supervisor of this behavior. *(Zucker, p. 61)*

14.

B. Borrowing medications can be dangerous. Report this information to your supervisor. *(Zucker, p. 61)*

15.

C. Report all side effects, no matter how slight, to your supervisor. *(Zucker, p. 61)*

16.

D. Changes in usual patterns of behavior may indicate a medication reaction. *(Zucker, p. 87)*

17.

B. Chemotherapy is the regimen of taking drugs to treat a malignancy (cancer). *(Zucker, p. 172)*

18.

D. Nail beds should be pink; this is normal. The other items are common reactions to chemotherapy. *(Zucker, p. 201)*

19.

B. When assisting with medications, be certain to ask, "Is this the right medication?" Check the medication list and label. *(Zucker p. 320)*

20.

A. Physicians and nurses are licensed to administer medications. The home care aide is not. *(Zucker, p. 319)*

21.

B. The home care aide is *not* licensed to administer medication. If you administer, you take all responsibility that goes along with giving medications. *(Zucker, p. 319)*

22.

B. Report to your supervisor if the patient does not know why he or she is taking drugs. *(Zucker, p. 320)*

23.

D. Medication reactions include skin rash, hives, and itching. Report these immediately. Intact skin is normal. *(Zucker, p. 320)*

24.

A. This is an appropriate action to assist with medications. The other items are considered medication administration. *(Zucker, p. 320)*

25.

A. You can assist patients as they take their own medications. *(Zucker, p. 319)*

26.

C. Many medications have similar names and look alike. Store these separately. *(Zucker p. 321)*

27.

C. Dispose of old medication so that no one else can make use of it or eat it by mistake. Do not put them in garbage or trash where children and animals may find them. *(Zucker, p. 321, Model Curriculum, p. 454)*

28.

C. Medications can be prescribed by a physician (oxygen) or obtained over the counter (aspirin and Tylenol). Juices are not considered medications. *(Zucker, p. 319)*

29.

C. All prescription medications should have information that relates directly to the patient, the medication, the pharmacy, and the physician prescribing it. *(Model Curriculum, p. 445)*

30.

A. Actually putting a pill into the patient's mouth is considered medication administration. Do not do this! *(Model Curriculum, p. 446)*

31.

A. Aspirin can cause bleeding in certain situations. Be sure the nurse knows that the patient takes any additional medication that is not on the list. *(Model Curriculum, p. 446)*

32.

B. Give gentle encouragement to patients to take their medications. *(Model Curriculum, p. 447)*

33.

B. The home care aide will not give the medications. *(Model Curriculum, p. 449)*

34.

C. Keep the medications in separate places to prevent the patient (and others) from taking the wrong medication. *(Model Curriculum, p. 449)*

35.

D. Patients should not be given the home care aide's home number. The other numbers, along with the number for the rescue squad, should be posted by the telephone for easy access. *(Model Curriculum, p. 450)*

36.

D. Misuse of drugs may develop intentionally or unintentionally. These are evidences of drug misuse. *(Model Curriculum, p. 451)*

37.

A. Drug dependency behaviors include failing to meet family or other important responsibilities. *(Model Curriculum, p. 451)*

38.

B. Petroleum jelly should not be used around oxygen. It is petroleum-based—a flammable material. *(Model Curriculum, p. 452)*

39.

D. The physician prescribes the medication, the pharmacist dispenses it, and the nurse may administer the medication. *(Zucker, p. 319)*

40.

B. Over-the-counter drugs can be purchased without a prescription. *(Zucker, p. 319)*

16 Simple Procedures

chapter objectives

Upon completion of Chapter 16, the student is responsible for the following:

➤ Describe how the home care aide changes nonsterile dressings.

➤ Define indwelling catheter.

➤ Identify external urinary drainage.

➤ Describe the role of the home care aide and intravenous therapy.

➤ Describe cast care.

➤ Describe ostomy care.

➤ Describe how the home care aide provides testing for glucose and acetone.

➤ Describe deep-breathing exercises.

➤ Identify how to make normal saline.

➤ Define sitz bath.

➤ Describe the role of the home care aide and hyperalimentation

DIRECTIONS Each of the questions or incomplete statements below is followed by four suggested answers or completions. Select **one answer** that is best in each case.

1. Which of the following types of dressing can the home care aide change?
   A. sterile
   B. nonsterile with medication
   C. nonsterile without medication
   D. all of the above

2. Which of the following statements best describes a dressing?
   A. a covering to protect the wound and the surrounding tissues
   B. a bandage to keep out pathogens
   C. a bandage to absorb drainage
   D. a covering to keep air and bacteria away from the wound

3. When there is drainage on the old dressing you are changing, you should:
   A. notify your supervisor immediately
   B. note the color, odor, amount and consistency on the chart
   C. refuse to change the dressing again without sterile gloves
   D. all of the above

4. When cleaning a wound, you should:
   A. wash your hands and put on gloves
   B. cleanse the wound in a circular motion from the clean area to the dirty area
   C. consider the wound clean and the skin dirty
   D. all of the above

5. In putting on a bandage, always:
   A. use sterile gloves
   B. hold it by the corners only
   C. tape completely around the edges
   D. all of the above

6. Which of the following would be best for throwing away a patient's dressing?

A. placing it in a trash can kept in the patient's bedroom
B. placing it in a trash can kept in the bathroom
C. placing it in a bag and taking to the outside trash can
D. placing it in a covered trash can in the kitchen

7. The term "ostomy" means:
   A. a temporary opening into the colon from the abdomen for the release of feces
   B. a permanent opening into the colon from the abdomen for the release of feces
   C. an artificial opening into the abdomen for the release of wastes from the body
   D. an artificially made opening which connects a body passage to the outside

8. A patient with an ostomy must wear an appliance to collect the matter released from the body. Which of the following is true about an appliance?
   A. Appliance bags can be permanent and must be cleaned, dried, and reused.
   B. Appliance bags can be disposable and must be thrown away after one use.
   C. Ostomy appliances are held in place with paste, adhesive, or a belt.
   D. all of the above

9. You can decrease the patient's embarrassment about an ostomy appliance by:
   A. understanding that it is usually a very traumatic event for the patient and be matter-of-fact when changing and cleaning the appliance
   B. keeping the area covered so that the patient does not have to see it when you are cleaning it

C. not allowing the family members to see it

D. all of the above

10. A ureterostomy is:

A. an opening into the ureter from the abdomen

B. an opening into the kidney from the abdomen

C. an opening into the bladder from the abdomen

D. all of the above

11. Your patient wants to know how long he will have his colostomy. Your reply should be:

A. "It is permanent."

B. "Just until the reason you had it made has been cured."

C. "This is something you must talk with your family about."

D. "I will ask my supervisor and then tell you."

12. You check your patient's colostomy appliance at 8:00 A.M. and then prepare and help her with breakfast. Her daughter comes to visit at 9:00 A.M. and complains because the bag is full. Your best response is:

A. "I can't do everything at once."

B. "It was not full when I checked it at 8:00 A.M."

C. "It is normal for her bag to fill after a meal."

D. "She did not tell me it had filled up since I checked it."

13. When changing an appliance bag and cleaning the area, you should:

A. allow the skin to dry thoroughly before applying new adhesive

B. use sterile bandages to wipe around the opening

C. use special soap to keep the skin from getting irritated

D. all of the above

14. The opening of the ostomy is called a(n):

A. ostae

B. stoma

C. ectomy

D. stotomy

15. Which of the following is/are needed in changing a colostomy appliance?

A. bedpan

B. disposable bed protectors

C. regular washcloth and soap

D. all of the above

16. When using a wafer around the opening of the colostomy, you should cut the hole:

A. the same size as the stoma

B. twice the size of the opening of the colostomy

C. half the size of the opening of the colostomy

D. 1/8 of an inch larger than the opening of the colostomy

17. Through which of the following ostomies would a patient receive nourishment?

A. ileostomy

B. ureterostomy

C. gastrostomy

D. colostomy

18. In cleaning your equipment after changing a colostomy, you would:

A. empty the wash basin into the toilet

B. flush the disposable appliance down the toilet

C. sterilize the bedpan

D. all of the above

19. Irrigating a colostomy is very similar to:

A. flushing a wound

B. giving an enema

C. changing a dressing

D. all of the above

20. When applying a cold compress, you must:
    A. not have ice directly on the skin
    B. remove it after 15 to 20 minutes
    C. cover the entire prescribed area
    D. all of the above

21. Using a hot water bag to ease aching muscles is a form of:
    A. moist heat
    B. dry heat
    C. moist treatment
    D. medication

22. Before applying a hot water bag, the home care aide should:
    A. cover it with a soft cloth or towel
    B. be sure that the bag is completely full
    C. be sure that the temperature is 180°F
    D. all of the above

23. Cold applications are used for all of the following reasons except to:
    A. reduce swelling
    B. reduce pain
    C. stimulate circulation
    D. stop bleeding

24. Important considerations for the home care aide who is weighing a patient include all of the following except:
    A. moving the scale frequently
    B. adjusting the scale as needed so the pointer is zero
    C. not holding onto the patient while he or she is standing on the scale
    D. recording the weight

25. A major concern in caring for a patient with a colostomy is:
    A. the skin condition around the stoma
    B. diet
    C. mobility
    D. concealing the appliance

26. When caring for a patient with a gastrostomy tube, the home care aide should:
    A. note the condition of the skin surrounding the tube
    B. remove the tube while bathing the patient
    C. administer tube feedings on schedule
    D. all of the above

27. When heat is applied to the skin, the blood vessels:
    A. narrow
    B. contract
    C. dilate
    D. constrict

28. Warm water is in contact with the skin. This is an example of:
    A. dry heat application
    B. local heat application
    C. moist heat application
    D. incompetence

29. The greatest danger associated with heat applications is:
    A. the possibility of burns
    B. increased blood flow to the site
    C. relief of pain
    D. improved appetite

30. Mr. Thomas has a hot water bag on his foot. You observe that his skin is pale. This means that:
    A. the hot water bag is working
    B. the hot water in the bag is not warm enough
    C. the hot water bag has been in place too long
    D. the hot water bag is too hot

31. When applying an ice bag, you should do all of the following except:
    A. place the bag in a flannel cloth cover
    B. fill the bag 1/2 to 2/3 full

C. use ice cubes to fill the bag

D. remove excess air from the bag

32. Which of the following is a dry cold application?

A. cold soak

B. ice bag

C. cold compress

D. cool water bath

33. A home care aide can change all of the following dressings except:

A. nonsterile

B. sterile

C. clean

D. thin film

34. Characteristics of drainage to note on a wound dressing include:

A. color

B. odor

C. amount

D. all of the above

35. You are to apply a clean dressing to a wound on your patient's arm. You should do all of the following except:

A. hold dressings by the corners

B. tape all edges of the dressing

C. assist the patient to apply any medicated cream

D. cleanse the wound and skin as instructed

36. An indwelling urinary catheter is inserted by:

A. the home care aide

B. the nurse

C. the family

D. all of the above

37. The urinary drainage bag should be placed:

A. on the side rails

B. at the level of the patient's bladder

C. on the bed frame lower than the patient's bladder

D. on the floor

38. The color of the urine draining into a drainage bag should be:

A. tea-colored

B. light to dark yellow

C. clear

D. red

39. Your patient has an indwelling (Foley) catheter and tells you that his bladder is full. You should:

A. report this to your supervisor

B. tell him that is normal with a catheter

C. tell him to urinate

D. raise the level of the drainage bag

40. The first step in catheter care is to:

A. wipe away from the meatus

B. wash your hands

C. tell the patient what you are going to do

D. position the patient on his or her back

41. The inability to control bowel movements or urine elimination is called:

A. incontinence

B. dehydration

C. diarrhea

D. constipation

42. Which of the following is *not* correct in providing perineal care for a patient with a urinary catheter?

A. Make sure the drainage bag is attached to the bed and that it is higher than the patient's bladder.

B. Always clean the perineum from front to back.

C. Make sure the tubing is not kinked.

D. Make sure the drainage bag and tubing are not touching the floor.

43. An external urinary catheter should be changed:
    A. every day
    B. every other day
    C. every 3 days
    D. once a week

44. When applying external urinary drainage, the home care aide may do all of the following except:
    A. position the patient on his back to expose the penis
    B. wash the entire penis and dry thoroughly
    C. roll the condom the entire length of the penis
    D. strap the condom on tightly

45. Intravenous therapy is:
    A. prescribed by a physician
    B. administered by the nurse
    C. changed by the home care aide
    D. A and B

46. The IV therapy line that uses veins in the upper extremities is called:
    A. peripheral
    B. central
    C. Groshong
    D. Hickman

47. IV catheters that have been surgically implanted into a large vein by a physician are called:
    A. peripheral lines
    B. central venous lines
    C. strategic lines
    D. peripherally inserted central venous catheters

48. An IV infusion in which the fluid and/or medication is always running is called:
    A. continuous infusion
    B. intermittent infusion
    C. peripheral infusion
    D. central infusion

49. A colostomy bag should be changed:
    A. when the patient is sleeping
    B. once a day
    C. when it is 1/2 to 2/3 full
    D. when odor is noted

50. The stoma area should be washed with:
    A. disinfectant
    B. alcohol
    C. oil
    D. soap and water

51. The adhesive ostomy device placed on the patient's skin around the stoma is called the:
    A. drainage bag
    B. wafer
    C. ostomy belt
    D. lubricant

52. Surgical openings into the abdomen through which a patient will receive nourishment include all of the following except:
    A. gastrostomy
    B. colostomy
    C. duodenostomy
    D. jejunostomy

53. Urine that has accumulated recently in the patient's urinary bladder is called:
    A. fresh
    B. new
    C. sediment
    D. acetone

54. Considerations with deep-breathing exercises include all of the following except:
    A. helping patients to inhale more air with less effort
    B. barrel chests are normal
    C. the goal is to change the patient's breathing habits permanently
    D. learning to deep breathe may be frightening to some patients

55. It is best to plan deep-breathing exercises:
    A. when visitors are present
    B. between mealtimes
    C. immediately after mealtimes
    D. late in the day

56. What is the first step in helping the patient with deep-breathing exercises?
    A. Offer the patient mouth care.
    B. Blow out through the mouth with lips "pursed."
    C. Document the activity.
    D. Breathe in deeply through the nose.

57. A solution of salt and water that is chemically very similar to the fluids in the body is called:
    A. Dakin's solution
    B. normal saline
    C. sterile water
    D. magic mouthwash

58. The area of the body that is bathed during a sitz bath is the:
    A. face
    B. chest
    C. perineum
    D. feet

59. The usual length of time for a sitz bath is:
    A. one hour
    B. 10 to 15 minutes
    C. 2 hours
    D. 30 minutes

60. To assist with hyperalimentation, the home care aide can
    A. mix the solutions
    B. allow the bottles to stand at room temperature at least 1 hour before use
    C. teach administration of the solution
    D. change the dressings on the catheter

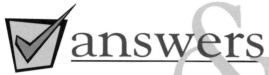

answers & rationales

1.

C. Sterile dressings with medications are usually changed by licensed nurses or those with advanced training in sterile technique and medication administration. *(Zucker, p. 325)*

2.

A. The type of dressing that is used will depend on the wound and the surrounding tissues. *(Zucker, p. 325)*

3.

B. These characteristics of drainage provide information about the condition of the wound and the healing process. Clean, not sterile, gloves are worn in changing nonsterile dressings. *(Zucker, p. 325)*

4.

D. All of these actions are appropriate in cleaning a wound. Use standard precautions. Clean in a circular motion to avoid contaminating already cleaned areas. The skin harbors bacteria that can infect the wound. *(Zucker, p. 326)*

5.

B. By holding the corners only, you do not contaminate the center of the dressings, which will go over the wound. Sterile gloves are not used for this procedure. Tape dressings in place, leaving the edges free. *(Zucker, p. 326)*

6.

C. Removing the dressing from the home decreases the chance for infection to spread. *(Zucker, p. 326)*

7.

C. An ostomy may release urine or feces from the body. Both are artificial openings made by surgery. *(Zucker, p. 336)*

8.

D. Ostomy appliances vary, so all of these statements are true. *(Zucker, p. 336)*

9.

A. A matter-of-fact approach helps to put the patient at ease. The patient and the family will eventually be responsible for the ostomy, so they should be involved in the care. *(Zucker, p. 336)*

10.

A. The ureter is a tube that drains urine from the kidney to the bladder. An opening into this tube is called a ureterostomy. *(Zucker, p. 336)*

11.

D. Some colostomies are temporary, and some are permanent. When you do not know the answers to questions, do not lie to your patient. Assure them you will get answers, and call your supervisor. *(Zucker, p. 337)*

12.

C. Eating stimulates peristalsis, which moves food through the digestive tract and brings about elimination. The patient cannot feel the bowel empty. *(Zucker, p. 109)*

13.

A. Adhesive will adhere best to dry skin, so the area should be dried thoroughly. It is not necessary to use special soap or sterile bandages when cleaning around the stoma. *(Zucker, p. 338)*

14.

B. The part of an ostomy that you see is the stoma, which looks like a pink rosebud. *(Zucker, p. 336)*

15.

D. All of these items are used in changing a colostomy appliance. *(Zucker, p. 338)*

16.

D. The opening must be large enough to slip over the stoma but not so large that feces can leak around the opening. *(Zucker, p. 338)*

17.

C. This is a surgical opening into the stomach that is kept open by a tube or screw cap. The patient receives all or part of his or her nourishment through this opening. The other choices are openings for waste products to leave the body. *(Zucker, p. 339)*

18.

A. The water in the wash basin is contaminated with fecal material and should be emptied into the toilet. Appliances are not flushable. *(Zucker, p. 339)*

19.

B. When you irrigate a colostomy, you wash out the large intestine with water. This is the same procedure that is used to give an enema, but the water is introduced through the anus instead of the stoma. *(Zucker, p. 339)*

20.

D. All of these actions must be performed. Cold compresses can decrease blood flow to an area, so they must not be applied for too long. Ice directly applied to the skin causes pain and vasoconstriction. *(Model Curriculum, p. 487)*

21.

B. Common forms of dry heat are the hot water bottle and the electric heating pad. *(Model Curriculum, p. 486)*

22.

A. Be careful not to let the plastic bag touch the skin directly, as it might easily burn the patient. The bag should be 1/3 to 1/2 full, at a temperature of 115° to 130°F. *(Model Curriculum, p. 486)*

23.

C. Cold applications slow the circulation to the immediate area, thus reducing swelling and pain and stopping bleeding. *(Model Curriculum, p. 487)*

24.

A. Moving the scale frequently may diminish its accuracy. *(Model Curriculum, p. 488)*

25.

A. Note the condition of the skin around the stoma and check for sores, redness, or anything that is uncomfortable to the patient. Report this to your supervisor. *(Zucker, p. 339)*

26.

A. Carefully observe the condition of the skin around the tube and report any changes. *(Zucker, p. 339)*

27.

C. Heat is a vasodilator—increasing the circulation to the area. *(Model Curriculum, p. 486)*

28.

C. Moist heat is when moisture is in direct contact with the skin. *(Model Curriculum, p. 486)*

29.

A. Burns, especially to fragile skin, are a real danger with heat applications. Observe and check the patient carefully. *(Model Curriculum, p. 486)*

30.

C. Pale skin beneath a hot water bag means that the bag has been there too long. Report this immediately. *(Model Curriculum, p. 486)*

31.

B. The bag should be filled 1/3 to 1/2 full with ice and water. *(Model Curriculum, p. 487)*

32.

B. The ice bag is a dry cold application. A cold soak, cold compress, and cool water bath are moist cold applications. *(Model Curriculum, p. 487)*

33.

B. Home care aides may not change a sterile dressing; this is done by the nurse. *(Zucker, p. 325)*

34.

D. Also note the consistency of the drainage. *(Zucker, p. 325)*

35.

B. Do not put tape completely around the edges of the bandage. *(Zucker, p. 326)*

36.

B. An indwelling urinary catheter is inserted by the nurse or the physician. It is a sterile procedure. *(Zucker, p. 327)*

37.

C. Never permit the bag to be on the floor! The bag may hang on the bed frame and must always be below the level of the patient's bladder. *(Zucker, p. 327)*

38.

B. It is normal for urine to change from light yellow to dark yellow, depending on the concentration and the amount of fluid the patient has consumed. *(Zucker, p. 327)*

39.

A. If the patient says he feels that his bladder is full or that he needs to urinate, report this to your supervisor. *(Zucker, p. 328)*

40.

B. First assemble your equipment, then wash your hands before proceeding. *(Zucker, p. 329)*

41.

A. An incontinent patient is one who cannot control his or her urine or feces. *(Zucker, p. 327)*

42.

A. The drainage bag should be attached to the bed frame and lower than the patient's bladder. *(Zucker, p. 328)*

43.

A. The external catheter should not be left on for more than 24 hours at a time and must be removed at least that often so that the penis may be washed and inspected. *(Zucker, p. 331)*

44.

D. Be sure the condom is secure—tight enough to hold the condom in place but not so tight as to hurt the patient. *(Zucker, p. 332)*

45.

D. Intravenous (IV) therapy is considered a medication; it is prescribed by a physician and administered by a registered nurse. *(Zucker, p. 332)*

46.

A. A peripheral IV line is placed in the upper extremities. *(Zucker, p. 332)*

47.

B. Central venous lines are IV lines in place, surgically, in large veins of the body. *(Zucker, p. 332)*

48.

A. A continuous infusion is uninterrupted; it is always running. *(Zucker, p. 332)*

49.

C. A colostomy bag must be changed when it is 1/2 to 2/3 full or when the adhering seal is broken. *(Zucker, p. 337)*

50.

D. The skin around the stoma can be washed with soap and water, just like the rest of the body. *(Zucker, p. 337)*

51.

B. A wafer must have a correctly sized opening, be secured around the stoma, and adhere snugly to the skin. *(Zucker, p. 338)*

52.

B. A colostomy is a surgical opening created to drain feces from the colon. The other ostomies are surgical openings for a patient to receive all or part of his or her nourishment and medications. *(Zucker, p. 339)*

53.

A. The word "fresh" is used to refer to urine that has accumulated recently in the patient's urinary bladder. *(Zucker, p. 342)*

54.

B. People who have had lung disease for a long time develop barrel chests, which are not normal. This is a result of extended periods of shallow breathing. *(Zucker, p. 343)*

55.

B. Because it also makes some people cough and bring up mucus, plan this exercise between mealtimes. This will minimize the potential for vomiting or loss of appetite. *(Zucker, p. 344)*

56.

D. After assembling equipment, washing your hands, asking visitors to leave, and telling the patient what you are going to do, you should direct the patient to breathe in deeply through his or her nose. *(Zucker, p. 345)*

57.

B. Normal saline has many uses because of its close chemical nature to the fluids of the body. *(Zucker, p. 345)*

58.

C. The patient sits in a special chair or tub with hips and buttocks in the water during a sitz bath. *(Zucker, p. 346)*

59.

B. Help the patient keep track of the time. The usual length of time for a sitz bath is between 10 and 15 minutes. *(Zucker, p. 346)*

60.

B. The other tasks are performed by licensed professionals, including the pharmacist and the nurse. However, the home care aide can assist by allowing the bottles to stand at room temperature at least 1 hour before use. *(Zucker, p. 348)*

17

Practice Exam

DIRECTIONS
Each of the questions or incomplete statements below is followed by four suggested answers or completions. Select **one answer** that is best in each case.

1. To whom should you report an incident or accident on the job?
   A. nursing supervisor
   B. physician
   C. your family
   D. patient

2. All of the following are examples of body language except:
   A. facial expressions
   B. touching others
   C. speaking
   D. hand movements

3. The home care aide participates in the development of the patient's plan of care by:
   A. writing the plan of care
   B. observing and reporting patient status
   C. obtaining physician orders
   D. all of the above

4. To provide security and consistency in caring for the patient with Alzheimer's disease, it is important to provide:
   A. sweets
   B. strict routine
   C. discipline
   D. frequent naps

5. Mr. Tucker has swelling in his right ankle. You know that he has chronic heart disease. You should encourage him to:
   A. remain in bed as much as possible
   B. elevate his foot as much as possible
   C. avoid walking and use a wheelchair
   D. drink lots of water

6. When caring for a patient with left-sided weakness, the home care aide should:
   A. perform all ADLs for the patient
   B. change the patient's schedule
   C. assist the patient to dress the left side first
   D. place food on the patient's left side

7. Activities of daily living (ADLs) are characterized as:
   A. physical needs
   B. cultural needs
   C. psychosocial needs
   D. spiritual needs

8. Reactions to pain include all of the following except:
   A. increased energy
   B. increased anxiety
   C. rapid pulse
   D. angry behavior

9. The traditional description of a female caregiver includes all of the following elements except:
   A. age 45 to 50 years old
   B. mother to her children, who are often teenagers
   C. wife to her husband
   D. caring for her siblings

10. Mr. Garren relies on his neighbor to help buy his groceries and his church members to take him to doctor appointments. This is an example of:
   A. family dynamics
   B. support systems
   C. disability
   D. culture

11. Mr. Tillman is a patient for whom you have cared 3 years. He just returned from a visit to the doctor, who told him that he had 6 months to live. Mr. Tillman says, "There

really isn't anything wrong with me." This is a reaction known as:

A. denial

B. anger

C. bargaining

D. acceptance

12. Characteristics of mental health include:

A. giving and accepting love and affection

B. anger, frustration, and anxiety

C. extended depression after losses

D. blaming others for one's disappointments

13. A patient who has feelings of extreme sadness—feeling dejected and discouraged— is experiencing:

A. aggression

B. denial

C. depression

D. projection

14. As you provide care and support to Mrs. Kline while she is being treated for clinical depression, you should report which of the following observations to your supervisor?

A. Mrs. Kline is able to feed herself.

B. Mrs. Kline refuses to take her anti-depressant medication.

C. Mrs. Kline assists with her bathing.

D. Mrs. Kline speaks to her sister on the phone twice a day.

15. Your patient tells you that he would like to die and has the gun to do it. Your response to this would include:

A. telling him not to talk like that

B. allowing him to talk about his feelings

C. demanding that he give you the gun

D. telling him that you don't blame him for wanting to end a life of pain and misery

16. When caring for a patient with a terminal illness who expresses concern about dying, the home care aide should:

A. tell the patient, "Everything's going to be all right."

B. listen and encourage the patient to share his or her feelings

C. change the subject

D. call your supervisor

17. One of the last functions to be lost is the sense of:

A. hearing

B. sight

C. taste

D. smell

18. After your patient dies, his family invites you to attend the funeral. You should:

A. decline because they are of a different religion than you

B. attend as your supervisor or schedule permits

C. offer to cook a meal for all participants

D. none of the above

19. Standard precautions are guidelines to be used:

A. in caring for patients with AIDS only

B. in caring for patients who are incontinent

C. in caring for any patient

D. only in the hospital setting

20. If you think the person in your care is not infected, you:

A. must follow standard precautions

B. don't have to wear gloves

C. don't have to change gloves between tasks

D. don't have to handle linens carefully

21. Oxygen therapy precautions include all of the following except:

A. monitoring the amount of oxygen in the tank

B. allowing the patient to smoke

C. checking the oxygen tubing for kinks

D. removing electrical appliances

22. Mrs. Brown has stacks of newspapers in a corner of her kitchen that are very old. You should:

    A. take them outside and burn them

    B. use them to wrap leftovers

    C. arrange for them to be given to a recycling facility

    D. move them to the basement

23. Which of the following foods is a high source of vitamins?

    A. chicken

    B. wheat bread

    C. eggs

    D. water

24. When buying foods that are high in protein, you can reduce the cost by:

    A. using red meat cuts

    B. using fillers such as bread crumbs or pasta to make a meat dish serve more

    C. using very tender cuts of meat for the elderly patient

    D. using beans and peas in limited quantity

25. Temperatures should be taken orally when the person is:

    A. on oxygen

    B. paralyzed

    C. alert and cooperative

    D. having trouble breathing

26. The term "vital signs" refers to:

    A. temperature, pulse, and respiration

    B. temperature, pulse, respiration, and blood pressure

    C. blood pressure, pulse, and respiration

    D. blood pressure, temperature, and pulse

27. Which of the following is a good principle of body mechanics?

    A. Keep your knees locked.

    B. Keep the person a few inches away from your body.

    C. Place your feet about 12 inches apart with one foot slightly ahead of the other.

    D. Twist your upper body as you lift.

28. Wrinkles in the patient's bed are uncomfortable and may cause:

    A. constipation

    B. itching

    C. bedsores

    D. incontinence

29. Mrs. Little is sitting in a chair while her bed is being made. The top linens are folded back so that she can get into bed. This is:

    A. an open bed

    B. a closed bed

    C. a surgical bed

    D. an occupied bed

30. After you have fixed Mr. Bell's breakfast, you return to his bedroom to find that he has fallen on the floor. What should you do?

    A. Stay with Mr. Bell and shout for help.

    B. Assist Mr. Bell to a chair and then call for help.

    C. Call your nurse supervisor for immediate advice.

    D. Assist Mr. Bell back into bed.

31. If a patient is undergoing a seizure, it is essential to:

    A. restrain the patient

    B. protect the patient from infection

    C. hold the patient's tongue down with your fingers

    D. protect the patient from physical injury

32. In an emergency, common first aid practices would include:

    A. moving the person from floor to bed

    B. leaving the person to get someone else to help

    C. controlling bleeding

    D. administering oxygen

33. When treating external blood loss, you should do all of the following except:
    A. apply direct pressure over the wound with a clean cloth
    B. if possible, elevate the limb to decrease the blood supply
    C. apply a tourniquet
    D. remain with the person until help arrives

34. You suspect that your patient has accidentally drunk some kitchen cleaner, and he is now unconscious. You should:
    A. give him a glass of milk
    B. position him on his back
    C. call for help and remain with him until help arrives
    D. induce vomiting

35. When providing mouth care for the unconscious patient, the home care aide should:
    A. rinse the patient's mouth with lots of mouthwash
    B. force the patient's mouth open if needed
    C. choose a toothbrush with soft bristles and rinse with lots of water
    D. position the patient's head to the side to prevent aspiration

36. When you help a patient with bathing and shampooing in a bathtub, check the water temperature with:
    A. your whole hand
    B. your elbow
    C. the patient's hand
    D. the patient's elbow

37. When the patient is using a shower, the home care aide should:
    A. stay with the patient
    B. check on the patient every 5 minutes
    C. have the patient call when finished
    D. leave the patient alone to bathe in privacy

38. When providing nail care for a patient, the home care aide may do all of the following except:
    A. cut the nails
    B. soak the nails
    C. clean with an orange stick
    D. file the nails straight across

39. When transferring a patient from a bed to a wheelchair:
    A. unlock the brakes of the wheelchair
    B. keep the bed flat
    C. position the wheelchair close to the foot of the bed
    D. place the wheelchair so that the patient will move toward the stronger side

40. When assisting a patient with a weak left side from a wheelchair, the home care aide should give support to the:
    A. weak side
    B. strong side
    C. front side
    D. back side

41. When helping a patient to stand, the first instruction the home care aide gives is:
    A. "Put one foot in under you."
    B. "Move to the front of your chair or bed."
    C. "On the count of three, push down with your arms, lean forward, stand up."
    D. "Put your hands around my waist."

42. Mr. Green has asked you to assist him to sit on the edge of the bed. The first thing the home care aide should do is:
    A. position your feet with a wide base of support and your center of gravity close to the bed
    B. tell Mr. Green what you are going to do
    C. roll Mr. Green onto his side facing you
    D. swing Mr. Green's legs over the edge of the bed

43. Patients who are bedbound are at greatest risk for:
    A. stiff joints
    B. bedsores
    C. bladder infections
    D. decreased appetite

44. Mr. Carter has diabetes. In providing his foot care, the home care aide should consider the following:
    A. Cutting toenails is permissible if requested.
    B. Feet should be soaked in water and bath oil for 5 minutes every day.
    C. Advise him to wear well-fitting shoes when out of bed.
    D. Dry, cracked skin is acceptable.

45. Places where obese patients are more prone to bedsores include:
    A. the outer thigh
    B. under the breasts
    C. the toes
    D. the ear lobes

46. Your patient has been saving medications for many years, and they are in her top dresser drawer. You should:
    A. throw all the pills away
    B. burn all the medications
    C. notify your supervisor
    D. encourage the patient to return them for a refund

47. Checking the name of the medication with the list of medications left by the nurse is assuring which right of medications?
    A. the right patient
    B. the right medication
    C. the right time
    D. the right amount

48. All of the following are considered medications except:
    A. oxygen
    B. aspirin
    C. Gatorade
    D. Tylenol

49. Which of the following is *not* correct in providing perineal care for a patient with a urinary catheter?
    A. Make sure the drainage bag is attached to the bed and that it is higher than the patient's bladder.
    B. Always clean the perineum from front to back.
    C. Make sure the tubing is not kinked.
    D. Make sure the drainage bag and tubing are not touching the floor.

50. It is best to plan deep-breathing exercise:
    A. when visitors are present
    B. between mealtimes
    C. immediately after mealtimes
    D. late in the day

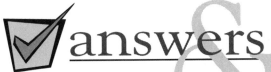

answers & rationales

1.

A. Your nursing supervisor is the person who is directly responsible for your activities. *(Zucker, p.12)*

2.

C. Body language gives silent clues to others about how you feel and what you want other people to do. Speaking is not silent! *(Zucker, p.17)*

3.

B. You are the health care team member who will spend the most time with the patient, so your observations are very important. *(Zucker, p. 22)*

4.

B. Follow the care plan carefully. The maintenance of a routine is one way to ease the care of the patient. *(Zucker, p. 366)*

5.

B. If an arm or leg is swollen, try to keep the part higher than the heart. Gravity will help the extra fluid to drain from the limb. *(Zucker, p. 180)*

6.

C. The involved or affected side is first into the garment and first out. *(Zucker, p. 205)*

7.

A. ADLs (e.g., bathing, grooming, eating) are best described as physical needs. *(Zucker, p. 30)*

8.

A. Actually, people in pain have increased fatigue, along with the other symptoms listed. *(Zucker, p. 33)*

9.

D. Most women caregivers are caring for a mother or father, who is 70 to 75 years old. *(Zucker, p. 36)*

10.

B. A support system is an arrangement that gives aid and comfort to a person. *(Zucker, p. 38)*

11.

A. Some people use denial when they meet a situation with which they cannot cope at the time. They say that nothing is wrong. *(Zucker, p. 39)*

12.

A. Giving and accepting love and affection is a significant characteristic of mental health. *(Model Curriculum, p. 180)*

13.

C. Depression is extreme sadness. The person feels dejected and discouraged, and it is shown by feelings of hopelessness, helplessness, and despair. *(Model Curriculum, p. 183)*

14.

B. You should report any change in patient behaviors, especially those that are detrimental to the patient's health. *(Model Curriculum, p. 186)*

15.

B. If you feel comfortable doing it, allow him to talk about such feelings while you listen patiently and caringly. *(Model Curriculum, p. 187)*

16.

B. Don't offer false hope or reassurance. Be a good listener, and encourage expression of feelings. *(Zucker, p. 88)*

17.

A. Hearing is the last sense to be lost. Talk openly and compassionately to a dying patient. *(Zucker, p. 90)*

18.

B. Some caregivers wish to attend the funeral of a patient. It gives them a formal chance to say goodbye and shows the family how much they cared for the patient. *(Zucker, p. 94)*

19.

C. Standard precautions are actions that are taken on a routine basis for all patients. *(Zucker, p. 121)*

20.

A. Standard precautions are actions that are taken on a routine basis for all patients. *(Zucker, p. 121)*

21.

B. Oxygen precautions include *no smoking*. *(Zucker, p. 153)*

22.

C. Do not keep piles of newspaper; they are a fire hazard. Arrange for recycling. *(Zucker, p. 152)*

23.

B. Grains are excellent sources of many vitamins. Meat, poultry, and dairy products are not. Water has no vitamin content. *(Zucker, p. 161)*

24.

B. This does make a meat dish go farther. Use poultry when it is cheaper than meat. Beans and peas can be substituted for higher-cost meats. *(Zucker, p. 166)*

25.

C. It is best for the patient to be alert and cooperative for you to measure oral temperature. *(Zucker, p. 271)*

26.

B. The term "vital signs" refers to blood pressure, pulse rate, respiratory rate, and temperature. *(Zucker, p. 269)*

27.

C. Placing your feet at least 12 inches apart provides a broad base of support and good balance. *(Zucker, p. 175)*

28.

C. Home care aides should make beds with no wrinkles in the sheets because they are uncomfortable and can cause bedsores. *(Zucker, p. 136)*

29.

A. The open bed is made when the patient is able to get out of bed and move around. *(Zucker, p. 143)*

30.

C. Contact your supervisor when any unusual event occurs. *(Zucker, p. 26)*

31.

D. Your role is to prevent the patient from injuring himself or herself. *(Zucker, p. 338)*

32.

C. Do not move the person unless he or she in great danger of further injury. Do not leave the person who needs help. Oxygen is not readily available as common first aid. *(Zucker, pp. 376–377)*

33.

C. Tourniquets are not used as first aid to treat external blood loss. *(Zucker, p. 383)*

34.

C. Expert medical help is essential. Stay with the patient. Do not give anything by mouth to the unconscious patient. *(Zucker, p. 384)*

35.

D. Turning the patient's head to the side prevents aspiration of any liquids into the patient's lungs. *(Zucker, p. 203)*

36.

A. First test with your whole hand, then permit the patient to check the temperature (to prevent the possibility of burning the patient). *(Zucker, p. 208)*

37.

A. Safety is a key point with all patient care procedures, yet you should provide as much privacy as possible without leaving the patient alone. *(Zucker, p. 211)*

38.

A. Home care aides should never cut the patient's nails. If the skin is accidentally cut, many patients are at high risk for infection or additional injury. *(Zucker, p. 209)*

39.

D. Utilize your patient's existing abilities, especially when transferring, for your safety and for the patient's safety. *(Zucker, p. 244)*

40.

A. Support the patient's weak side, permitting him or her to freely use the strong side and assist with the transfer. *(Zucker, pp. 179, 244)*

41.

B. The sequence begins with instructing the patient to "move to the front of the chair or bed." This gets the patient closer to you for safety and proper body mechanics for both of you. *(Zucker, p. 243)*

42.

B. Inform the patient what you intend to do, how you intend to do it, and how he or she can assist. *(Zucker, p. 240)*

43.

B. Bedsores, or pressure sores, are areas where the skin has broken because of pressure. Bedbound patients are a great risk for bedsores. *(Zucker, p. 193)*

44.

C. The proper shoes are well fitting and give support. Going barefooted is not advised. *(Zucker, p. 196)*

45.

B. Obese patients tend to develop bedsores where body parts rub together, causing friction, such as under the breasts, between the folds of the buttocks, and between the thighs. *(Zucker, p. 193)*

46.

C. Some elderly patients save medications that become outdated and then start taking them again. The home care aide can help to maintain safe medication practice by notifying the supervisor of this behavior. *(Zucker, p. 58)*

47.

B. When assisting with medications, be certain to ask, "Is this the right medication?" Check the medication list and label. *(Zucker p. 317)*

48.

C. Medications can be prescribed by a physician (oxygen) or obtained over the counter (aspirin and Tylenol). Juices are not considered medications. *(Zucker, p. 316)*

49.

A. The drainage bag should be attached to the bed frame and lower than the patient's bladder. *(Zucker, p. 324)*

50.

B. Because it also makes some people cough and bring up mucus, plan this exercise between mealtimes. This will minimize the potential for vomiting or loss of appetite. *(Zucker, p. 343)*

Index

Answer Sheet

You may make additional copies of this answer sheet as needed.

Directions:
1. Fill in only one circle, using a number 2 pencil.
2. Keep all marks inside the circle.
3. Blacken the circle completely.
4. Completely erase any answer you wish to change, and make no stray marks.

1 Ⓐ Ⓑ Ⓒ Ⓓ Ⓔ   26 Ⓐ Ⓑ Ⓒ Ⓓ Ⓔ
2 Ⓐ Ⓑ Ⓒ Ⓓ Ⓔ   27 Ⓐ Ⓑ Ⓒ Ⓓ Ⓔ
3 Ⓐ Ⓑ Ⓒ Ⓓ Ⓔ   28 Ⓐ Ⓑ Ⓒ Ⓓ Ⓔ
4 Ⓐ Ⓑ Ⓒ Ⓓ Ⓔ   29 Ⓐ Ⓑ Ⓒ Ⓓ Ⓔ
5 Ⓐ Ⓑ Ⓒ Ⓓ Ⓔ   30 Ⓐ Ⓑ Ⓒ Ⓓ Ⓔ
6 Ⓐ Ⓑ Ⓒ Ⓓ Ⓔ   31 Ⓐ Ⓑ Ⓒ Ⓓ Ⓔ
7 Ⓐ Ⓑ Ⓒ Ⓓ Ⓔ   32 Ⓐ Ⓑ Ⓒ Ⓓ Ⓔ
8 Ⓐ Ⓑ Ⓒ Ⓓ Ⓔ   33 Ⓐ Ⓑ Ⓒ Ⓓ Ⓔ
9 Ⓐ Ⓑ Ⓒ Ⓓ Ⓔ   34 Ⓐ Ⓑ Ⓒ Ⓓ Ⓔ
10 Ⓐ Ⓑ Ⓒ Ⓓ Ⓔ   35 Ⓐ Ⓑ Ⓒ Ⓓ Ⓔ
11 Ⓐ Ⓑ Ⓒ Ⓓ Ⓔ   36 Ⓐ Ⓑ Ⓒ Ⓓ Ⓔ
12 Ⓐ Ⓑ Ⓒ Ⓓ Ⓔ   37 Ⓐ Ⓑ Ⓒ Ⓓ Ⓔ
13 Ⓐ Ⓑ Ⓒ Ⓓ Ⓔ   38 Ⓐ Ⓑ Ⓒ Ⓓ Ⓔ
14 Ⓐ Ⓑ Ⓒ Ⓓ Ⓔ   39 Ⓐ Ⓑ Ⓒ Ⓓ Ⓔ
15 Ⓐ Ⓑ Ⓒ Ⓓ Ⓔ   40 Ⓐ Ⓑ Ⓒ Ⓓ Ⓔ
16 Ⓐ Ⓑ Ⓒ Ⓓ Ⓔ   41 Ⓐ Ⓑ Ⓒ Ⓓ Ⓔ
17 Ⓐ Ⓑ Ⓒ Ⓓ Ⓔ   42 Ⓐ Ⓑ Ⓒ Ⓓ Ⓔ
18 Ⓐ Ⓑ Ⓒ Ⓓ Ⓔ   43 Ⓐ Ⓑ Ⓒ Ⓓ Ⓔ
19 Ⓐ Ⓑ Ⓒ Ⓓ Ⓔ   44 Ⓐ Ⓑ Ⓒ Ⓓ Ⓔ
20 Ⓐ Ⓑ Ⓒ Ⓓ Ⓔ   45 Ⓐ Ⓑ Ⓒ Ⓓ Ⓔ
21 Ⓐ Ⓑ Ⓒ Ⓓ Ⓔ   46 Ⓐ Ⓑ Ⓒ Ⓓ Ⓔ
22 Ⓐ Ⓑ Ⓒ Ⓓ Ⓔ   47 Ⓐ Ⓑ Ⓒ Ⓓ Ⓔ
23 Ⓐ Ⓑ Ⓒ Ⓓ Ⓔ   48 Ⓐ Ⓑ Ⓒ Ⓓ Ⓔ
24 Ⓐ Ⓑ Ⓒ Ⓓ Ⓔ   49 Ⓐ Ⓑ Ⓒ Ⓓ Ⓔ
25 Ⓐ Ⓑ Ⓒ Ⓓ Ⓔ   50 Ⓐ Ⓑ Ⓒ Ⓓ Ⓔ